Long Term Care Administration

About the Author

Ben Abramovice has been a leader in the field of aging and long term care for over 5 years. He is currently the administrator of Laguna Honda Hospital, the largest municipally-owned long term care facility in the country; a multi-level, diverse organization that renders both institutional and non-institutional long term care services. Dr. Abramovice has taught long term care administration on a graduate level for many years, and has been involved in legislation and public policy for over two decades. He was a participant in both the 1971 and 1981 White House Conference on Aging. Dr. Abramovice brings to this field of education diverse personal involvements in virtually every aspect of the long term care continuum. He has held membership and offices in different professional organizations including past President of the California Association of Homes for the Aging, member of various committees on the House of Delegates of the American Association of Homes for the Aging, and a presenter at numerous professional gatherings. Considered one of the most original thinkers in the field, Dr. Abramovice has written a text directed primarily for the future administrator in long term care. While the focus of his text is on undergraduate health administration education, the book will be invaluable for entry level graduates, practicing professionals, and people who need familiarization on aging and long term care.

A graduate of UC Berkeley, Dr. Abramovice has his Masters and Doctorate in hospital administration from the University of Chicago and Columbia Pacific University, respectively. For the past six years he has led Laguna Honda Hospital into becoming one of the nation's outstanding long term care facilities.

More recently he has lectured in China, under the auspices of the Shanghai Public Health Department, and has established a sister facility relationship between Laguna Honda and the Haudong Hospital in Shanghai. He has visited and lectured at different long term care services throughout eastern and western Europe, and has been a consultant to numerous organizations on issues connected with long term care.

This marks the first text by Dr. Abramovice, and we understand that several other professional books are in the process of being written.

Long Term Care Administration

Ben Abramovice, MBA, PhD

The Haworth Press
New York • London

The Haworth Press, Inc., 12 West 32 Street, New York, NY 10001
EUROSPAN/Haworth, 3 Henrietta Street, London WC2E 8LU England

Library of Congress Cataloging-in-Publication Data

Abramovice, Ben.
    Long term care administration.

    Bibliography: p.
    Includes index.
    1. Long-term care facilities—Administration. 2. Continuum of care. I. Title.
RA999.A35A25 1987   362.1'6'068   87-11949
ISBN 0-86656-399-7

CONTENTS

Foreword

For those of us who have labored long and hard in the field of Long Term Care, Ben Abramovice's book is akin to water sluicing over parched earth. While we have not lacked for articles, seminars, position papers and conferences all of which have addressed pieces of the long term care puzzle, a seminal text which brings all the pieces together in a comprehensive way has until this time been absent.

I am pleased to say, upon reviewing *Long Term Care Administration* that the drought is over. Whether you are a seasoned administrator, a rookie in training, a Director of Nursing, geriatric social worker or a long term care physician, this book should be required reading.

For starters the author views long term care in its broadest sense. Although he is a nursing home administrator, he shows an acute awareness of the interrelationship between nursing homes, home health agencies, hospitals, hospices and other institutions along the health care continuum.

Secondly, as a veteran manager of long term care facilities he is well aware that no one individual or profession can administer in a vacuum. The text addresses the multiple roles of everyone from the head of maintenance to the facility administrator, with excellent discussions around the nurse aide and the dietary department. Those of us who believe in the team approach to service delivery owe Dr. Abramovice a debt for so clearly setting out the collaborative process.

Lastly and perhaps most importantly in this era of rapid change, the text sets out in clear detail the various models of service delivery from the much maligned medical model to the current panacea, the psychosocial model. Whether the reader intends to manage a 100 bed non-profit facility or a 300 bed proprietary facility, he will find not only food for thought, but concrete suggestions on what action to take under what set of circumstances. One cannot ask more of any text.

So be you student, planner, policymaker, nurse, administrator or consumer, like that famous beer "this book's for you!" It is a blueprint for those who wish to become successful long term care managers and an invaluable resource to those who are already seasoned administrators.

Paul Kerschner

Preface

The evolution of this text has taken many years; a whole career, I may say . . . On many occasions in the past decade, I have started to write about the administration of long term care facilities, only to find that the "facility" had changed, making my presentation obsolete. Or, I would find that the system had changed so much that I was actually telling more about less by focusing on the administration of a long term care institution.

The recognition that things were changing so fast was in itself a revelation. That which had been static for so many years was now dynamic and changing. It was important for me to understand the phenomena as much as it was for me to formulate a plan to deal with the new demands that would develop in this field.

In my early years as a consultant in the field, I was particularly concerned with design, construction and the operation of the nursing home. This exclusivity itself made me uneasy, because I was fully aware that the nursing home, as it was operated in the 1960s, was not "long term care" in the true sense, but the most visible component of a whole array of services that existed even in those days. This tunnel vision, not unlike the affliction that possessed legislators and other policy makers, retarded the development of the long term care system as we now envision it. Educators were also in the same trap, but even in worse shape. Academia had virtually ignored long term care in any significant dimension. I remember writing a paper in 1960 describing the relationship between the nursing home and the acute hospital. In it I described the "poor cousin" role the nursing home played at its very best. The relationship of this so-called black sheep of the health family to the acute hospital has changed little in the 25 years since I wrote that article. The field itself, however (especially in the last three or four years), has developed dramatically. With this change came my own personal reawakening of interest in doing a definitive book in this field, and the state-of-the-art at present. I recognize that such an attempt would probably still be caught on the cusp of the dynamics of change, and at some short time after its publication could be considered out of date. I felt the risks were worth the effort and consequently wrote this text acknowledging the state of flux the entire long term care system is currently in.

In describing what this text is, it may be important to point out what it is not. First of all, it is not a cookbook to administration. There are no easy formulas or recipes for success; nor is it a didactic reiteration of regulations with the illusion that following regulations will also guarantee good patient care, patient well-being or good quality of life. None of these, of course, would be true even if I claimed it to be so.

Also, although I tried, this is not a definitive textbook. Much more could be done in certain specific areas, such as public policy, management style, community organization, and so on. In essence, therefore, this is not a traditional textbook, but a phenomenological approach to education. It is being written as a undergraduate textbook, to be an adjunct for health and human service administrative programs. It is also designed to satisfy the needs of the new graduate student, who has little or no experience in the field, as well as an office reference book for the practicing professional in long term care.

The undergraduate will find this textbook designed for relatively easy integration with most other health or human service administration undergraduate programs. With luck and the proper utilization of this textbook, a whole generation of health and human service administrators will be released upon the population with some reasonable knowledge about what is, in actuality, one of our country's largest human service systems.

Again, this is not a cookbook, nor does it offer formulas for guaranteed success. It is a distillate of experiential administrative practice throughout my career, and to the extent that my own successes have outweighed my failures, the student will benefit.

I would like to acknowledge the constant support given me by Dean Bill Winston. His encouragement allowed me to persevere and ultimately finish this text, while maintaining an uncommonly demanding work schedule. I would like to thank Diane Seiler, my secretary, who organized the "putting together" of this text, and stuck with the project, contributing her very practical knowledge of organization in a very important manner. Dave Counter's contribution in Management Information Systems was very helpful, and many thanks to Jonathan Goldman, Loren LeJeune and Philip Alonso for their secretarial assistance.

WHO WE SERVE

Since we have chosen a resident centered management approach, it behooves us to study the nature of the clients that we will serve. First of all the very entitlement of this group of individuals may be important. Traditionally if they are in a health facility, they are called "patients"; if they're not in a health facility they may be called other things, such as "client." If it's an adult day health or home care situation, "participant" would be appropriate; while a health-related facility would house "residents." There is a trend to call the recipient of services (some are even called "recipients") by names that do not relate to degrees of sickness or the pathology of their cases. We tend to be disinterested in terms that represent the acute hospital or the medical model; the idea being that we're discussing a life space or "biosphere" of a person rather than their medical history.

It should be recognized that what the population served is called often reflects the mentality of the people that govern that service. To the extent that that mentality defines the paradigm of that service, we should understand these terms and their significance.

RESIDENT-ORIENTED DECISION MAKING

It is at great risk that we attempt to design this textbook as a study guide for "administrators focusing on resident needs." Not that that isn't the goal of all health administration, but too often that phrase is used as a platitude. The very "Mom and apple pie" statement that "administration is resident-oriented" obscures the fact that most administration is really system-oriented and facility-oriented; and very often the idea that "what is good for the institution is good for the resident" prevails. Decisions made on a daily basis, or decisions of great importance can always be "rationalized" as being "resident oriented." Yet, on close scrutiny, one cannot make the link between any individual resident benefit and the decision being made. In order to be able to forge a more direct link between the decisions made in LTC and the betterment of the life of the resident, we must know much more about the resident, his needs, wants and desires, than we usually do. We must also know the demographics of the population-at-large and a variety of other elements that contribute to the long term care system in its current form. This is not to say that decision making with the facility's, or the system's, greater purpose in mind is invalid, inappropriate or unethical; quite to the contrary. What we are saying is that when we make a decision we should have very clear in our minds if it is a resident oriented decision, an institution oriented decision or in all honesty something self-serving for the professional network that serves the elderly. We will not rationalize the many types of self-serving decisions we often see in health administration, but attempt to look positively at a full range of decision-making modalities. Our intention is to increase their relativity to the residents' well being. To the degree that decision making, ethics, and resident needs are all intimately linked, we will have a chapter on ethical considerations. At this point we will dwell on the needs of the long term care recipient as defined by the needs of the population as a whole.

ACUTE AND LONG TERM CARE COMPARISON

We may now ask why the administrator of a long term care service needs to know so much about those they serve, while a person in a comparable role in an acute setting may not need that degree of insight.

At the outset we must recognize that the long term care administrator is in a qualitatively different ballgame. The long term care administrator is, by and large, working in relatively small organizations and the normal management barriers that separate the direct delivery of service and management are virtually nonexistent. While the administrator in an acute hospital has many layers separating him from "where the action" is, the administrator of a long term care service finds himself totally immersed in all aspects of the operation. Another and even more important reason for the long term care administrator to understand and know the population that he serves, is because that knowledge will govern his decision making process. The long term care administrator has the luxury of being able to define his population with some degree of clarity, whereas the acute administrator must deal first with the full spectrum of health needs of a variety of segments of our population. This specificity warrants special attention and we must spend some time on not only describing this profile on a variety of levels, but attempting to relate them in this and subsequent chapters, to the function of the administrator.

THE AGING PHENOMENON

As a starting point to understanding the needs of the elderly population, we should review certain theories connected with the aging process. The understanding of these theories and their implications directly relates to the management of appropriate delivery of services.

THE DISENGAGEMENT THEORY

In the early '60s the "disengagement theory" as evolved by Cumming and Henry described a process of withdrawal of the aging individual from society and of society's concurrent withdrawal from that individual's life sphere. This theory suggests that the withdrawal is associated with changes in goals, attitudes and orientations of the older person. It describes the "biosphere" as a constricting space in which a curtailment of involvement is experienced. The theory extends this idea to suggest that society equally disengages from the aging individual and that this is a healthy and beneficial process to both society and the individual.

The disengagement theory was generated from the study of a relatively limited group of individuals who were reasonably healthy and not deprived. Unfortunately, this concept was accepted by many segments of our society including those groups that made public policy. People found that this theory supported their own viewpoint in terms of its application to the institutional setting. In the early '60s (as we noted) the institutional component of the long term care system was beginning to become a dominant force in our health care system. The acceptance of this theory not only by public policy makers, but by different groups of public health professionals and administrators, condoned the inattention to the social needs of the institutionalized person and fostered and augmented the mentality that created row upon row of somambulant disabled elderly sitting in wheelchairs lining the wards and hallways of both state hospitals and newly emerging private sector nursing homes. A common defense against this form of benign neglect was to pull out a slightly distorted summary of the disengagement theory and justify what were, in fact, dehumanizing conditions. Soon, however, there were many challenges to this theory that rationalized the exclusion of the elderly from the mainstream of our society.

Arnold Rose offered a countering theory that the elderly—being excluded from society for a variety of reasons—formed their own subculture, creating a peer-integrated group linked by common interests, problems and activities. The suggestion this theory makes is that the elderly benefit most by their own age-integrated social milieu. If public policy makers and developers of programs for elderly take this theory to heart, they would view its tenets as quite supportive of age-segregated housing, and of the historical trend of removing the elderly to their own communities, more or less outside of the mainstream of society. In this context, the term "subculture" must be viewed as pejorative, especially in defining a "group" as large as the elderly.

Another theory—somewhat more positive—has been called the "activity theory," which calls for augmented socialization and social integration and stresses "recreational" formats of activity programming. This, of course, is a theory that supports the idea of recreational programming in institutional and non-institutional settings, such as the traditional bingo, birthday events and crafts.

A subsequent theory called the "developmental" or "life cycle" theory emphasizes the unique evolution that individuals have, and places the responsibility for aging on the enlightened individual. This individual should—consistent with the "do your own thing" mentality of the '60s and early '70s—provide his/her own standards and develop through the life cycle by personally developed guidelines. If one were to accept this as the theory of aging, we would leave the elderly to their own devices, and not engage in the social and (in a broader sense) institutional responsibilities of problem solving, program developing or broad stroke planning. The next social view of aging relates to what may be called the symbolic "interactionist" view of aging, which incorporates the environment and all elements of that environment as they impact on the person. Changes in the variety of stimuli inherent in the individual's environment are most significant in this context, and a variety of behavioral characteristics, such as depression, dissatisfaction, low self-esteem, are viewed as products of environmental interactions that occur. An administrator could cull from this approach to social aging, the positive concept of designing a managed environment, which will be discussed in a later chapter.

When we see how significant interventions are in the environment of the elderly institutionalized person, strong support can be made for this concept of aging. If this concept can be transferred to the home of the individual who receives support services, or to the adult day health care or to any of the other elements of the continuum, we can see how currently significant an understanding of the symbolic interactionist view of aging can be.

While all of these theories seem to have flaws, a total concept of long term care management could be created from the more acceptable elements of each concept. What one finds in the context of any group of recipients, whether they be a group of people receiving home meals or institutionally-bound elderly, is that certain of the characteristics from these theories are represented very clearly. Therefore, in order to administrate your service properly, not only should these theories be understood, but their most useful elements can and should be extracted to help formulate operating policy.

Criticisms of these somewhat formal theories of aging have centered primarily around the negatives they suggest. It is my contention that the "kernel of truth" contained in each can be used in a most positive manner: not merely for the purpose of administering and designing service delivery functions, but on an even broader level in the development of successful public policy.

BIOLOGICAL FACTORS IN AGING

For the sake of completeness, we must also understand the variety of key theories in the biological aging process. We can utilize this theoretical information to better understand the group dynamic that governs the reaction of our resident or client population. The theory that aging is primarily a genetic mechanism predominates with cellular aging being governed by genetically derived chromosomal elements. The relationship between the genetic aspect and the environmental aspect of aging will never be stated with any degree of surety in the near future. But suffice it to say that whether the theorists of aging claim the environment or the genetic-inherited characteristics as the more important component in the aging process, both views have substantial amounts of empirical information available in their support.

Concurrent with the traditional biological/environmental approach to aging are a variety of sub-issues relating to very specific components of aging, such as, for example, cellular oxidation—biochemical variables that may thwart the aging process or enhance the immune system to prevent aging processes. Many times in the practice of administration, you will find that your clients adhere to one or another "trendy" mode of preventing aging, and each year brings us new utilizations of medicines, vitamins, poultices, and metaphysical stratagem to prevent the aging process. Certainly there is only one alternative to aging—death—which does not seem to be acceptable to most parties. It is most important, in the light of these client concerns, that the administrator be able to understand both the social and biological aging theories, in order to recognize their implications for successful delivery of service.

AGING CHARACTERISTICS

Regardless of how you interpret or utilize theories of aging, certain characteristics of the aging process directly relate to your management schema. As our society changed from a rural agrarian society to an urbanized industrial society, the role of the elderly person both in the culture and the family changed significantly. Whereas in an agrarian society the elderly has an historically-defined role and function in the family unit, none was created for the elderly person in the industrial society. In point of fact, our society neatly excluded the elderly person from the family and the labor force by not only not having designed their functional role in either sector. Consistent with this evolution of technology came the construction of homes that did not allow for space for the elderly generation, and the consequent change of the elderly's position in the family from asset to liability. Rapidly changing technology accentuated the lost role of the elderly in the household by making his knowledge less relevant to the knowledge currently needed to survive and thrive by the younger entrants to the society. The acceleration of technology and its impact on the elderly is clearly seen today, where very few older people are able to pass on, in a genuine and traditional manner, their experiential knowledge to the younger generations.

Concurrent with this loss of functional role in the family and the loss of their status as both breadwinner and a transmitter of knowledge was the loss in the dignity that these other characteristics bestowed upon them. What we see, therefore, is a pattern of multiple psychic losses in the process of aging that must be understood in order for us to operate as effective managers in the LTC system.

What we have been talking about has been social loss. Concurrent with these is the reality of diminished sensory capabilities that is part of the biological aging process. While scientists may disagree on the extent to which elderly suffer sensory loss, it is generally accepted that sensory capacity diminishes (at different speeds) in later years. For example, while hearing loss may be the first noticeable sense to decline, feeling may be the last. The sense of taste decreases so that by the age 80 possibly over 50% of the tastebuds are gone and therefore sense of taste has to be redefined for this age group. The sense of smell lingers on, as does the sense of feel. Due to changes in the physical structure of the eye, vision also undergoes a regression in later years.

Collectively the sensory losses directly relate to the individual's ability to perceive and cope with his/her environment. If we as administrators of services to the elderly recognize these diminished capabilities, we can utilize that information to address the need for supports within the environment to counteract sensory deprivation.

This level of understanding of the needs of the elderly is imperative to successful administration of the service, whether institutional or non-institutional. A significant step in the qualitative enhancement of the life of the service recipient is the acceptance of responsibility by the administrator to offset the social and physical losses we've just described. While this subject will be discussed further in the section on managed environment, I must emphasize that this approach varies substantially from the traditional perception of administrative management, which relates primarily to traditional fiscally-oriented management and organizational training. A resident-centered approach, however, is pivotal to the administrator's ability to succeed in delivering quality service and enhancing quality of life for the recipient.

CHARACTERISTIC HEALTH CONSIDERATIONS

Current thought in the field of aging does not consider the process of aging to be a disease. The normalcy of the aging process as genetically determined (with environmental aspects factored in) contradicts the theory that aging is a disease process. While certain major diagnostic categories are currently being viewed as a disease process (Alzheimer's) the non-pathological viewpoint of the aging process seems to be most widely supported. While there are diseases that are characteristic of the elderly population, by and large they have health problems that are not unlike the total spectrum of our society. Given that there are variations in immune system response, absorption capabilities of the gastro-intestinal tract and other age related variables, there is no intrinsic reason for the elderly to be a sicker component of the population than other components. This viewpoint being stated, we must also acknowledge that the elderly occupy and account for close to a third of all acute hospital days although they represent approximately 12% of the population. This gives rise to the misconception that the elderly are basically an illness ridden population. Other factors such as the large number of medications used by elderly and allegedly high costs for care, confuse the health profile of the elderly considerably.

We must recognize that the majority of the elderly are relatively healthy, and that only about 5% need skilled nursing beds. Another 17% need some form of protective living environment, be it senior housing or residential care, both of which will be discussed in future chapters.

As we move through the '80s we are able to see the senior health picture with greater clarity. In the context of training for long term care administration, we will be able to define health needs with more accurate specificity. With this increased level of specificity we will be able to offer health programs comparable to those offered the rest of the population—of a preventive nature and utilized to defer disability and counteract those regressive cycles that are commonly part of the aging paradigm.

There are, however, three forms of psychosocial problems that appear more evident in the older population than with the population at large. They are depression, paranoia and hypochondriasis. For a nonmedical person sometimes a little bit of information can be dangerous. The individual can generalize from a very limited base and make wrong conclusions. Acknowledging this I hope this information can be utilized very directly in improving your administrative ability to serve your elderly recipient. These very common medical phenomenon in the elderly should be understood but used with great caution. Certainly one must not pigeonhole all our residents into 1 of these 3 categories! This could lend to a grave misunderstanding of the aging phenomena. Use this information rather as VERY BASIC guidelines for behavioral problems that *can* be responded to from the administrator's desk.

For example, assume that a person's visual and auditory problems contribute to his/her uncertainty about the environment. If their glasses are broken or improperly prescribed, the distorted environment then may serve as a stimulus for suspicion. Perhaps we can better understand our own impression that this person is paranoid. Equally, if a person can't hear properly, communication becomes indistinct, and it is easy for that individual to hear whispers and other distorted communication. This increases, again, a sense of suspicion of the environment, based, in this case, on hearing loss. By the same token, if hypochondriasis or abnormal concern with the body's functions and responses is understood by staff, they can then address the needs of the resident much more appropriately. To carry this to conclusion, if we realize that a large percentage of frail elderly and particularly institutionalized elderly have sub-clinical depressions caused by a number of factors, we can also conclude that these depressions can be "treated" by non pharmaceutical techniques.

A positively designed environment with good stimulus, supportive communication and a variety of other elements can go a long way to reduce these depressions, and, in many cases, totally reverse them; thus reducing the need for medication (which is often considered the only solution for these conditions).

The essence of this discussion as it relates to the management is that the administrator has a great deal of control over that which happens in the institution above and beyond pure medical service delivery. The environment, the training of the staff, the creation of appropriate stimulus, the development of supportive activities are all concerns and responsibilities of the administrator. It is quite possible, therefore, through appropriate management of the long term care service (institutional and non-institutional) that those negative or clinical characteristics often attributed to the elderly can be modified, and that the nursing home in particular can become a health giving, positive, wellness oriented environment.

HISTORY OF LONG TERM CARE

Aging by a significant percentage of individuals in a population is a relatively new historical phenomena. Until recently, there was no noticeable aging population for many reasons. Disease, poverty, famine and war prevented many people from reaching old age. In addition, elderly and disabled individuals who did survive were not separated from the non-elderly who had a variety of mental and physical disabilities. People who displayed various kinds of anti-social or "immoral" conduct during segments of the Post-Reformation period were also lumped with the elderly, and the mentally and physically disabled.

The English Poor Laws of the early 1600s were a major step in recognizing the existence of these needy populations and creating some form of societal solution to the problems that this body of people posed for the developing societies. These laws relegated those individuals who had no other support to almshouses, and they were the model utilized by colonial America for dealing with the limited, but ever-present minority of elderly and disabled people and the larger number of able bodied poor. As early as the late 1600s almshouses were built in Boston through application of these English Poor Laws.

We cannot exclude from this discussion the historical relationship of the Church to the health care of the day. Through medieval times health care was a function of the church. Hospitals as they were then configured, offered limited, if any, services to the elderly disabled. If one were to study England at the beginning of the industrial revolution, one would note that both the church, private philanthropy, and parish-supported almshouses were the primary givers of the "institutional" care of the day for the elderly, disabled and all others. One view would be that this form of service is charitable, but the sharper observer might suggest that the burgeoning population of "undesirables" cluttering the expanding urban environments of these newly-industrialized western societies was offensive to the emerging middle class. It was probably as important to rid from public view the sight of these poor unfortunates as it was to render them humane and charitable services.

With the emergence of the industrial societies, the idea that the elderly and disabled should be removed from public view because they were deemed undesirable became firmly entrenched—this despite the fact that at this time there was no significant population of the aged that could be distinguished from the overall population of unfortunates benefiting from these "services."

Certainly as the agrarian societies of the west shifted to industrialism, the function within the family of the honored elder changed, and the value of the elderly within the family unit diminished. The respect accorded the aging agrarian for his knowledge of the land and as a transmitter of oral traditions was lost in industrial society.

In this country in the early 19th century, the widespread existence of almshouses and poor farms, and the emergence of church and fraternal organizations that aided the elderly and disabled, descended directly from the first steps taken by European nations three hundred years earlier to cope with a new population of "undesirables."

Even during this later period, there was still no exclusivity given to the elderly although by this time industrial society was generating a growing population of urban elderly. Toward the middle of the century, however, we began to see two systems of serving this population. Specifically, one —governmental implemented through the county poor farm and almshouse; and the second—non-governmental and charitable—implemented through religious, ethnic and fraternal organizations. For example, many homes for the aged, such as Hebrew Home for the Aged and Disabled (currently known as the Jewish Home for the Aged) and the Women's Benevolent Society Home were started in the late 1800s.

The impact of the philanthropic organizations, which served their particular membership only, was slight. The bulk of the service rendered to the elderly was via the poor farm almshouse approach, and abuse of these unfortunates is legendary. Although reforms were attempted at different points in the 18th and 19th centuries, the interests of the elderly were a very low priority, especially when set against the impact of the immigration of hundreds of thousands of Europeans to this country in the late 19th to early 20th centuries. These masses of new Americans would prophetically enough form the bulk of the aging population that would finally have to be coped with by the mid-century.

While medical technology expanded in the early part of the 20th century, the aged and disabled housed in county farms or nonprofit homes for the aged were still at the bottom of the totem pole when it came to treatment. The concept, started years before, of removing these people from the mainstream, was embraced by a mentality that governed the developing field of medicine. The historical attitude of "putting away" an "undesirable" population begun in the early years of industrialism has plagued the elderly and the disabled to this day.

During the first three decades of this century medical care evolved from a system of individual practitioners who rendered services in their patients' homes to a hospital focus where resources were concentrated, and emphasis was placed on the short term acute medical services. This, of course, further alienated the aged and chronically disabled who could not share in the positive aspects of this centralizing of medical care delivery.

It was not until the depression in the early 1930s that a large elderly disabled and now indigent population emerged. Not only were there no economic benefits for them, but certainly those that found themselves in an institutional setting had no health benefits, which had already been limited before the economic crisis. The country was now also feeling the effect of the aging of the immigrant population, a phenomenon which for 4 or 5 decades to come would be a significant factor in the delivery of services to the aging population. American society, in the mid-30s was experiencing the developed impact of many forces: immigration, industrialization, one-family housing, and a lack of any economic safeguards against the plunge into indigency and despair. At the same time, the increase in hospital-based medical practice further removed the needy who lived in residences for the aging from any hope of significant medical attention.

The primary nature of the facilities that housed the elderly during this period was that of a residential care home or boarding home. The people initially living in these homes were, in relative terms, healthy. As time went on, however, the body populace became older and sicker, and these non-health institutions added more services in order to deal with the emerging medical reality in the populations they served. A similar approach was taken by county farms (county poor houses) that began as residential care establishments. As their population aged and became more chronically ill, they added nursing services. This metamorphosis was encouraged by new laws that offered economic inducement to institutions who cared for the medically needy. But because of the isolation (if not exclusion) of these institutions from the mainstream medical establishment there was no linkage between the newly evolving hospital system and what we may call the precursor to the current long term care system.

The passage of the Social Security Act of 1935 was a milestone in that an insurance mechanism, old age survivors insurance (OASI), was the first significant effort of the government in support of the elderly. It paid primarily for what amounted to boarding home care, and therefore increased the demand for (and ultimately supply of) these facilities, which tended to serve a more affluent population. Another component of this legislation, under Title I, was the OAA, or old age assistance. The depression had forced many owners of large homes to convert these homes and take in elderly boarders. Thus, we see the precedent for the conversion of private residential facilities to boarding homes which ultimately became part of the nursing home system that existed in the '50s and early '60s. Since these facilities were still not part of the medical care system, and the new programs spawned by the Social Security Act of 1935 were not medical in nature. By 1940, there were approximately 1200 facilities designated as nursing homes with a total bed count of 25,000. Governmental regulations for these facilities, were, in essence, non-existent.

By the early '40s, therefore, we find we have three systems of the institutional component of long term care: the charitable nonprofit, composed of religious, ethnic and fraternal facilities serving (in most cases) distinct populations; the governmental, or public sector, which maintained poor houses and county farms for the indigent; and the recently emerging boarding home/nursing home, many of which were newly funded by the OASI or the OAA cash assistance programs, and which catered at that time to a private paying clientele.

The '40s was a decade characterized by a quantum leap in the development of medical technology. This war-driven explosion in medical care created an even greater gap between the long term institutional care system and the acute system. Ironically, however, this very division created some very positive relationships between the two systems.

During the '50s the nursing home, was considered—at least in schools of hospital administration—as a part of progressive patient care. Unfortunately it was also considered the *end* of progressive patient care, in that when the acute care system could no longer successfully cure or remedy a problem, the concept of progressive patient care relegated that individual to the nursing home. During the '50s these homes were no different in substance from those in the '40s in that many were converted residences. It was not until the latter part of the '50s that the demographics of the aging population began to make a major impression on government policy makers.

By 1960 the elderly population had grown to 16.7 million. This was a considerable jump from the 6.7 million elderly in 1930. Another important factor in initiating legislation was the perceived shortage in hospital beds, and the contention that the elderly were occupying valued short term care beds when they could be cared for equally well in long term nursing beds. To deal with the pressure created by the bed shortage, hospitals began to utilize the services of nursing homes as part of what they were calling progressive patient care. This relationship was not necessarily designed to serve the needs of the aged as much as it was to make beds available for people who had a better economic base for their care.

In 1960 the passage of the Kerr-Mills Bill was the first major incursion of the federal government into the support of the medical needs of the elderly population. This further encouraged the expansion of the nursing home system.

The developing interest in funding medical assistance for the aging led to the 1961 White House Conference on Aging, where the specific needs of the elderly were defined with great clarity. To this point, there had been no clear definition of a nursing home. As a matter of fact, a nursing home was defined as any facility in which a majority of its residents received some form of nursing care. It would surprise many that in the Kerr-Mills (MAA) there was no statutory definition of skilled nursing. It was not until about 1964 that a semblance of definition which related to the need for licensed personnel at a set number of hours per week, evolved.

With the emergence of the MAA program, the number of nursing homes grew 127% between 1961 and 1964. There was still, however, no more than a minimal linkage between nursing homes and the acute care system.

In 1965 the most important social legislation to date supporting an individual's rights to receive medical care was embodied in a Medicare and Medicaid legislation. Medicare, a health insurance, and Medicaid, a welfare program, were directed primarily at the aged and the poor. Incorporated in the body of this legislation were fiscal incentives for the additional expansion of the institutional nursing home system. The reimbursement formula contained inducements to attract capital, and the lack of a highly structured regulatory process allowed the possibility of profitability because of a laissez-faire regulatory approach.

These laws also demonstrated the first effort on the part of the government to regulate and define services. These regulations and definitions were of necessity derivative of the acute hospital system, already regulated by government agencies and controlled by law. It was a logical next step to attempt to design the nursing home as a mini-acute hospital. Therefore, the terminological definitions of service and specifications of physical plant were all derived from the acute hospital standards. Though one of the intentions of this legislation was to reduce skyrocketing hospital costs by making less costly alternatives available and attractive, in practice the laissez-faire regulatory system emphasizing acute related technology raised LTC patient costs in nursing homes to record levels.

Two new terms were coined; ECF, extended care facility, and skilled nursing facility (SNF). The "extended" in extended care proved to be a misnomer (or at least improperly perceived), because it did not refer to the provision of care over an extended period of time, but rather to the provision of active treatment as an extended hospital care. The idea was to provide lower cost care for people who still required general medical management and skilled nursing on a continuous basis—but who did not need the high technology and doctor-intense environment offered in an acute hospital.

In 1967 public law 90-248 established an intermediate care facility with the intention of shifting as many as 50% of the recipients of skilled nursing home services to these types of facilities. But this program has not been functional, and after an initial spurt of growth, both the idea and practice of an intermediate care facility system fell into dormancy. Concurrent with this legislation in 1967 were minimum standards of functioning for skilled nursing facilities and in 1972 the legal distinction between the ECF and the skilled nursing facility was removed.

By the early 1970s public outcry over the poor conditions in nursing homes spread throughout the country. Many states conducted hearings, and by 1975 a high percentage of states incorporated federal law with state law, bringing about the highest regulatory standards thus far seen in the long term care system.

Between 1964 and 1974, as the nursing home "industry" boomed, hundreds of thousands of nursing home beds were constructed. Towards the middle of the '70s the rate of growth slowed, and by 1980, growth in expansion terms of the total number of beds was minimal. From this point in mid-decade, the institutional component that represents the nursing home field is very close to saturated (although, depending on geographic characteristics, there are areas where there are now more available nursing home beds than would be expected).

Throughout the decades since 1950, changes have occurred that have made the long term institutional long term care system dominantly proprietary. Approximately 70% of all nursing home beds in this country are proprietary. The public sector, which for many years was the predominant form of serving the institutional needs of the elderly, has decreased in both absolute number and percent of the entire long-term care system. Few, if any, public sector long term care beds have been constructed, and in many cases wards and facilities have been closed down.

The nonprofit private sector composed of religious, ethnic and fraternal organizations showed a growth period between 1965 and 1975, but it still plays, in terms of size, a subordinate role to the newly emerged proprietary component of the system.

The nonprofit private sector, which will be described in future chapters has its own distinct characteristics.

Another trend that began in the mid-'70s was the emergence of large corporate entities absorbing existing single sole proprietor ownership of nursing homes. At present, a high percentage of all nursing home beds are owned by corporations or nursing home chains that have two or more facilities in their organization.

Thus far we have spoken only of the brick and mortar components of the long term care system. Throughout the period described, though, there were many attempts to serve elderly people outside of the institution. During the '30s programs to attract people to center locations were started on the East Coast. Throughout the ensuing decades, home care, senior centers and the variety of non-institutional programming operated on the fringe of the very diffuse isolated long term care institutional system. The 1971 White House Conference on Aging expanded the Administration on Aging to deal with all of the needs of the elderly population. Specifically, it encouraged the development of non-institutional services in a much more comprehensive fashion than ever before. Among the results of the evolution of an administration on aging were the creation of local area agencies linked statewide and federally, and the emergence of federally funded nutrition programs to act as focal points for the gathering of the elderly and the frail elderly. Other movements for the development of an integrated system of institutional and non-institutional service began during the seventies as a reaction against perceived abuses in the nursing home delivery system. By the White House Conference of 1981, it was recognized that the population of elderly was in the neighborhood of 25 million and that services at levels previously unconceived were needed to serve the health and social needs of this very large—and growing—part of the American population.

CONTINUUM OF CARE

The continuum of care that we are describing is not continuity of care as it is taught in the schools of hospital administration nor is it progressive patient care as described in many health administrative textbooks. Rather it is a view of the elderly person in the context of an organized system of services needed to prevent regression, to encourage maximum independence and social and physical functioning. These services should be linked in a logical pattern and available at the right time, at the right place, and in the right quantity.

A final standard for the continuum of care is that it must be economically feasible for the elderly person.

HOME

The continuum of care as described in this text uses as a starting point the home of the frail elderly. Use of the word home often conjures up the quaint cottage and the white picket fence. Let us expand on this definition of home in more realistic terms. Very rarely since the 1930s were homes constructed to allow adequate space for the elderly in the family home as was common during the agricultural or agrarian period in our history. When we talk about the elder's home, we may not be meaning that house owned by the elderly person. We may be describing one of the following alternatives.

SINGLE ROOM OCCUPANCY (SRO)

This term describes commercial hotels and rooming houses usually in city central that serve the urban poor or transient populations of our cities. The elderly form a substantial core of this population. Also included in this category are residential hotels and smaller rooming houses. This inexpensive housing, which may serve in excess of 400,000 elderly at this time, is out of the mainstream of the planned housing system. Because of this, it is subject to the whims and fancies of the local government in their efforts to redevelop deteriorating neighborhoods. Most often, however, this form of housing stock has no place in planning for the long term needs of the elderly.

CONTINUUM OF CARE

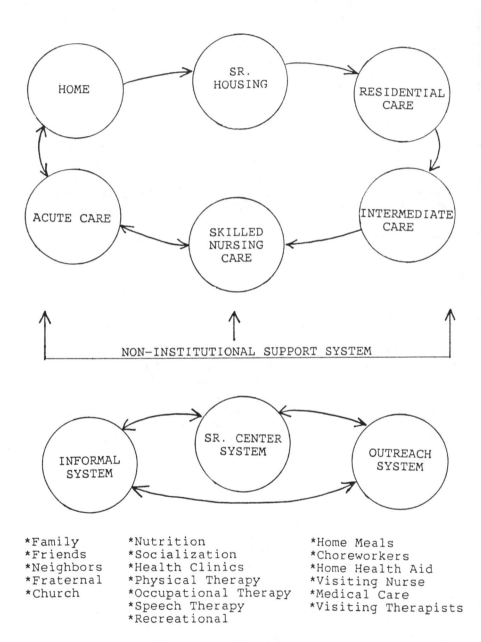

*Family   *Nutrition   *Home Meals
*Friends   *Socialization   *Choreworkers
*Neighbors   *Health Clinics   *Home Health Aid
*Fraternal   *Physical Therapy   *Visiting Nurse
*Church   *Occupational Therapy   *Medical Care
                     *Speech Therapy   *Visiting Therapists
                     *Recreational

FOSTER HOMES

A very limited number of elderly are housed in residences with several other non-related people. These foster homes are designed to create a small extended family under the observation of the owner of the home. Foster homes differ from boarding homes in that the individual participates in the life of the "family" and offers greater participation in the community. Under these conditions there is a greater involvement in the community by the frail elderly. The foster home concept is quite limited and studies have been done to determine the direction in which this small sub-system should go and/or to evaluate it in respect to the entire system.

MISCELLANEOUS HOUSING OPPORTUNITIES

We have the opportunity at this point to mention age-old methods of caring for the elderly, such as "granny cottages" or "granny flats." This allows a form of semi-independent living, since these structures are usually in the backyard or very closely tied to the main house. Add-on apartments are part of the same concept. These forms of housing reduce stress caused by the anticipation of relocation and provide privacy while allowing for the existence of an informal support network to be close at hand.

EQUITY CONVERSION

We should recognize that on many occasions, the home is no longer acceptable because of the fact that the elderly individual may be cash poor and unable to maintain the house properly. This lack of money to support the house has forced many people to go into a protective environment prematurely. Equity conversion allows a person who is cash poor to convert this equity for living expenses, emergencies, chore service or personal care. Equity conversion has certain risks for the elderly person, and if nothing more, may impact on that individual's wish to leave an estate to their kin. Equity conversion, of course, is a time limited factor, since when the equity is utilized, a movement is forced with little or no resources left to the individual. At any rate, it is a concept that is currently gaining popularity since more people are reaching maturity with home owner status.

The Elderly at Home

For the sake of this particular discussion we are addressing the frail elderly. We could just as easily start the continuum with the needs of the healthy elderly person, for there are many. Using the frail elderly as a starting point however gives us a common denominator in terms of service needs that can be defined with outcomes that have some degree of predictability. When we describe the elderly at home it could be a private home, an apartment, a downtown hotel, a granny cottage, or a room in one of their children's homes. We are also making the assumption that the elderly person benefits by being at home and that our efforts to help her retain a high level of independence and functioning capability will be applied to maintaining her there.

Whether this is a tiny room with a toilet down the hall, or a spacious mansion, the definition of assessed needs will be the same. As we learned from our description of the client population, loneliness, isolation, depression and physical regressions are part of the profile of a large percentage of elderly people.

INFORMAL NETWORK

The primary system that maintains the nation's frail elderly is the informal system, composed of family, neighbors, churches and fraternal group support. It is said that up to 70% to 80% of our elderly currently utilize this support system. In rural areas it is much more visible than in urban areas where isolation and loneliness are such an integral part of city living. The informal network is the most interesting and complex of all the systems in the continuum. Some believe that its success is due to its lack of structure, lack of professional input, or of government involvement. Another viewpoint, however, is that to make the informal network work maximally, training and organizing of these resources is necessary. Consequently, there have been many efforts to train these informal "caregivers" in the rudiments of care. Family members and neighbors can be trained to give hands on care in assisting the frail elderly in dressing, bathing and grooming. Certainly volunteers from the neighboring church can be used to assist in shopping or cleaning the elderly person's home. To the degree that this kind of support system is intrinsic to rural living, the lack of the volitional support system in urban areas could be countered by some structuring and organizing by appropriate community organizations. There are many examples of the church being used as a training site or as a senior center. There are examples of fraternal groups such as the Lion's Club or Oddfellows forming transportation pools for the elderly to transport them to doctor visits, shopping or recreational activities. These organizational elements of the informal network can often be enhanced and encouraged to function in a structured way with appropriate professional administration and guidance. There are ways to coordinate this network effort even though it may be spread throughout the community.

SENIOR CENTER SYSTEM

If our continuum is to be effective, we should address the needs of the individual at the point where she is still mobile enough to leave home to receive certain support services. In order to do this we will develop a construct called the senior service center. A variety of specially designed programs are offered the elderly who come to this center. The center's primary emphasis is socialization, and its ability to attract the elderly encourages mobility. The senior center as a discrete entity offers its services with the intent of preventing the psychologically regressive cycle that will inevitably face the seniors if wholly left to their own devices. The center may offer a wide range of support services under a single roof: communal dining; medical screening clinics for diabetes; blood pressure; heart, podiatry clinics; legal consultation services; and assistance with dealing with governmental programs, such as social security; and many others. The senior center, with its multiplicity of services is a vital first link in the continuum of care, and a cornerstone for the successful development of the other components of the continuum.

The senior centers can either be a "freestanding" or part of the facility such as a hospital, nursing home or governmental building. In concept, however, regardless of the physical housing of the service center, it is viewed as separate and distinct from the home or whatever other brick and mortar combinations the elderly live in.

Financial Considerations

Most senior centers are administered by individuals who have come from the fields of social service and have worked their way into this with no distinct training or defined curricula for this kind of administrative work. Yet because of the proliferation of senior service centers, their increased complexity and their great importance to the success of the rest of the continuum, it is imperative that a structured, well-trained management emerge as a guiding force.

The primary source of funding for senior citizen service centers throughout the country is Title 3 of the Older Americans Act, which funds senior nutrition sites throughout the country, and supplies adjunct funding for the many kinds of services currently seen at these centers. Although—again—the primary purpose of the senior center is one of socialization, a strong emphasis should be placed on nutrition and a variety of paramedical support services.

OUTREACH SYSTEM

The third major system in the continuum is the outreach service system. Its primary role is to keep the elderly person independent and functioning maximally as he or she begins to lose the degree of *mobility* that allows a trip to the senior center, or a visit with the family or a shopping trip. Loss of mobility due to motivational or physical factors in itself breeds regressive circumstances.

As reduced mobility affects the elderly individual's life, outreach services offer the support needed to prevent the regressive cycle. Usually the first request for service emerges around the individual's inability to properly shop and cook for himself. Or perhaps additionally she is no longer able to clean her apartment properly. The service most commonly provided from this outreach system is that of homemaker or housekeeper, also called sometimes a choreworker. The choreworker would shop, clean house and cook. It is possible there might be no need for additional services beyond this level. Empirically we find, however, that the next stage of regression finds the individual afflicted with memory loss and unable to acceptably perform toileting, dressing and grooming functions.

Additionally, the elderly person might be unable at this stage to self-administer prescribed medication. The next service, therefore, that this system can offer is a home health aide trained in rendering hands on service. This aide is able to assist in dressing, bathing, toileting and grooming, and should have the training to do relatively simple health-oriented services, such as range of motion, administration of certain kinds of drugs, and minor treatments as prescribed by a physician.

As physical regression increases, more medically sophisticated services may be needed, such as a visiting nurse, visiting therapists, physicians, and so on. In conjunction with their apparent needs for nutritional support, the outreach service system would also be able to supply a home meal (known in many areas as "Meals on Wheels"). The socializing visit in this program may be as important as the nutrition components of the food.

Other possibilities for outreach services may include the need for legal services, social services, and creative art programs, to name but a few. In sum, the outreach service system implies a separate non-institutional base that provides services to elderly who are unable either to perform these services for themselves.

Here again we find a service system without a homogeneous organizational structure. Administrators evolve normally from one of the para-medical services, such as nursing or physical therapy. As we've discussed in the senior center system, there is a need, if the system is to survive, to have a more formalized educational program that will allow maximum effective management to make these systems operative.

There are two services that exemplify the center concept and the outreach concept. We will explore these more thoroughly at this time.

ADULT DAY HEALTH CARE

Adult Day Health Care as currently constructed is one of the most significant elements in the long term care continuum. Its essence is the offering of certain specialized services to non-institutionalized frail elderly that will help support them in a relatively independent setting. While adult day health care could be offered to people in residential care settings, most of the people who are appropriate recipients of this service are either living at home or in senior housing.

Adult day health care utilizes and relies heavily upon an in-depth assessment of the applicant's needs. (The individual who receives service may be labelled a client or a recipient.) The services rendered by adult day health care include all of the traditional rehabilitative services, such as occupational therapy, physical therapy, speech therapy, plus an array of medical, nursing and paramedical services that are combined into specially designed programs for each recipient. The paramedical services will include nutritional, social services, pharmaceutical, and a variety of other services brought in on an as-needed basis.

The referrals to adult day health care may come from a variety of sources, including families, physicians, social workers and discharge planners. The assessments are normally done by a member of the staff of the adult day health care and then evaluated by a multidisciplinary team that develops a special treatment plan or program for each individual. This will consist of a certain number of full-day visits per week and specialized programming with the context of these visits. Normally adult day health care will have its own transportation system to pick up the frail elderly person and bring her to the day care site.

Because of the incomplete continuums that exist in most communities and the fact that one service, normally skilled nursing predominates in the continuum, inappropriate placements are sometimes made into nursing homes. It is believed that the enhancement of the adult day health care system will allow people to remain at home longer by receiving these intermittent day care services, and thus prevent inappropriate or premature institutionalization. The day care center may choose the level of service it wishes to render on the basis of a variety of factors. If it is designed properly it will meet the demand of the community it serves, and therefore the level of service will be determined by that community demand. On the other hand, the level of service may be defined by the intrinsic economics of the day care center: most centers throughout the country are marginally financed and require grants, community support and a variety of configurations of "soft money" to survive.

Recently there have been some experiments with adult day health care centers based in proprietary skilled nursing homes, but the results of these model projects are not available as yet.

One of the issues in adult day health care is whether the service should be institutionally based or free standing. There are many arguments for and against each of these viewpoints. It also depends on what kind of institution you are discussing, because proprietary nursing homes, nonprofit homes for the aged, and acute hospitals have all attempted to offer adult day health care. Each of these services have different economic structures. From an economic standpoint alone, one must look much further than just the terminology of "institutional-based services."

On the other side of the coin, those people who feel adult day health care should be rendered on a non-institutional or community basis, have data to support the economics of that approach.

The management of adult day health care usually consists of a director (who is normally a registered nurse), clerical support, a professional staff consisting of direct caregivers, and an ancillary support staff for transport, hands-on patient assistance, and clerical back-up. The most important function of the adult day health services in the continuum of services is its central position in the network of non-institutional care. Because of this strategic location, linkages with home health, nutrition and other support services can be rendered easily, as well as appropriate and supportive ties established with institutional-based service deliverers.

The administrator of an adult day health care center should be qualified on the master level in a field closely related to human services. My own preference is that the administrator of an ADH be a registered nurse. I think the training and work experience of most registered nurses would lend itself to appropriate staffing patterns and a good understanding of the monitoring and service delivery of the ADHC. A registered nurse, with a graduate degree in some form of health management would be entirely appropriate. I feel strongly that the education must be heavily directed toward administration and management. Ultimately, the success or failure of an ADHC will rest more on administrative ability than on programmatic or clinical abilities. This is probably true of most administrative positions in long term care. In ADHC, the administrator shall be responsible for program and budget. The administrator will also be responsible for any licenses and regulatory controls. An administrative plan which would include an organizational chart is a good first step. Recruitment, employment, training of new staff and assuring that manpower will be adequate to meet the needs of the program are also among the responsibilities of the ADH administrator. Circumstances may warrant administrative responsibility for two centers. Further expansion of the administrator's authority should be done only with a clear understanding of the governmental bodies that license, certify or regulate the service.

The next administrative person at the ADH facility is the program director, who shall be professionally qualified in either nursing, social work or human services (recreational, occupational or physical therapy). This individual should have demonstrated a competence at working with the impaired elderly person. It is perfectly legitimate for the administrator to also be the program director, if the administrator has these professional qualifications and time for additional responsibilities. The responsibility of the program director is the development of a program appropriate to recipient needs. This means implementation and co-ordination of the program, the evaluation of the program recipients' changing needs, and the initiation of corresponding program modifications. The program director also is involved in supervising employees and volunteers.

The third person in the organizational structure at the ADH facility is the activity co-ordinator, who should be a person appropriately trained in direct service to disabled elderly. Most appropriately the activity co-ordinator will be trained as an occupational therapist, art therapist, music therapist or recreation therapist. A social worker could also be considered qualified, with appropriate experience. The activity co-ordinator will be responsible for the development of the part of the program designed to encourage self-care, prevention of mental and physical deterioration, and the resumption of normal activities for the recipient.

Some specific duties of the activity director would be the assessment of each client's interests and needs, and the development, based on this information, of a personalized activity program. This includes the recording, dating and periodic (quarterly) monitoring of each recipient's progress. The activity director also will supervise program aides and other activity workers, and be responsible, as mentioned above, for co-ordinating the entire program of activities as it relates to the group as a whole.

Other members of the ADHC service include nursing, occupational therapy, physical therapy, psychiatric (and psychological) services, medicine and nutrition. Since a major thrust of the ADHC program is to maintain or improve proficiencies in the activities of daily living, the occupational therapist will use his skills to train or strengthen muscles and nerve functions, and will suggest any modifications to the participant's home environment that may be necessary in order to accomplish the end of successful independent living. Skilled nursing service, is supplied by a registered nurse, is needed to assess particular needs for personal care, and assist in the more ordinary activities of daily living, such as toileting, bathing, grooming, and eating. Additionally, skilled nursing provides health education and counseling to both participant and family. Nursing will administer medications and treatments as prescribed by the physician and provide, if necessary, training in self-administration of medications and treatments. Supportive and restorative nursing care will be delivered at the day care site. It should be remembered that the nurse is a valued part of the multi-disciplinary assessment team, and not only does her work contribute to the overall care plan, but her observation, monitoring and documentation form a core service upon which other observations and components of the care plan are built.

Psychiatric and psychological consultations are usually done by independent contractors for a certain specific number of hours per week. These professionals contribute their assessment of the participant as a component of the participant care plan; other members of the multi-disciplinary team will observe, monitor and re-evaluate the effect of their recommendations. A psychiatric social worker or a psychiatrically-trained nurse could, with appropriate experience, fulfill the function of psychiatrist or psychologist on this multi-disciplinary team.

The Medical Social Worker

The medical social services shall focus on interviewing and screening potential users of the service to determine how appropriate ADHC would be for the applicant. They would also be responsible, to a great extent, for referring those people who are inappropriate for the ADHC to some other service that would be in their best interest. The social worker also contributes to the counseling needs of the participant and would be very active in the referral to and discharge from the ADHC program, and in referral to available community resources when the need for ADHC is no longer evident. The social worker would also be involved in assisting the multi-disciplinary team in interprofessional dealings. The social worker should also serve as a liaison with the participant's family, home and neighbors, and may even link the participant more closely with other community organizations or components of the informal network, such as church, fraternal or neighborhood organizations. This latter responsibility shall include, if possible, linkage to in-home support services, home nutritional services, and the ongoing monitoring of the recipient's needs.

Nutrition Services

It is advisable that a professional dietitian be employed, at least on a part-time basis, to ensure appropriate therapeutic diets and nutritional consultation for each individual participant. At ADHC a noon meal will offer at least one third of all recommended daily dietary requirements. As part of the nutrition service, the dietitian will provide counseling and education, and will be an active participant in the multi-disciplinary team. With their help, the dietitian will monitor, maintain, and evaluate the effect of the nutrition services.

Multidisciplinary Team

In describing the modus operandi of the ADHC, we see a very fine example of the use of the multi-disciplinary team, which most health-oriented services attempt to do. In the case of ADHC, it is mandatory for the survival of the day care organization. The successful co-operation and interweaving of the input of a variety of professions will aid immeasurably in determining how successfully the recipient responds.

In each aspect the professional input must be complete with documentation, monitoring, periodic assessments, evaluation and change. The program director, who is usually the facilitator of the care plan development, must be responsible for modifying views and assuring that there is balance in the care plan.

Physical Therapy Services

The physical therapist should be a registered physical therapist (RPT). Their function is to relieve pain and develop or restore functions, using a variety of modalities, such as massage, heat and sound, exercise. Some of the kinds of programs offered by physical therapy would include therapeutic exercise, gait training, massage, prosthetic training, and a variety of other rehabilitative services.

Occupational Therapy

To expand on our previous definition of an occupational therapist, the occupational therapist would attempt to increase the capability for independence and enhance the physical, emotional, and social well-being of the recipient. Therapeutic, creative and self-care activities all will be part of the occupational therapy program. Programs of a diversional nature—leatherwork, weaving, ceramics and graphic arts—will also play a role. A variety of programs would maximize sensory stimulation and co-ordination exercises, concentrating on the more successful utilization of the upper extremities. Beyond that, there might be training in the use of adaptive equipment for the activities of daily living, such as feeding and dressing and bathing. These are but a few of the approaches commonly used by occupational therapists.

Speech Therapy Services

The speech therapist will not only develop and implement plans for appropriate speech and language therapy, but work with family and friends to help them assist the recipient in correcting speech disorders.

Medical Services

The staff physician of an ADHC service will develop the medical component of the care plan, which will include the authorization for medication, treatment, special nutritional programs, OT, PT and speech. To some degree the physician "legitimizes" the work of the paraprofessionals in a process similar to that which would take place in an institutional setting. If the patient's own primary physician assumes responsibility for the program implementation at the ADHC, that physician should then be responsible for the same functions that the day care physician would normally provide. The dialogue between the physician on the ADHC staff and the recipient's primary physician should not be confused by a replication of responsibility. Sometimes difficulties are caused when the primary physician feels his responsibilities are being usurped; this easily can be avoided by the proper integration of services at the start. A set policy and procedure should clearly describe the relationship between the primary physician and the day care physician.

In addition to the administrative and professional staff we have just described, volunteers, case aides and paraprofessionals should be used in numbers adequate to the need for their services. Properly trained paraprofessionals will allow greater use of limited professional time. We must remember that the funding for these services (primarily through the Medicaid program), is very limited, and it is important that the per diem cost for these services be tightly controlled. The use of these paraprofessionals and volunteers can reduce the use of higher cost licensed or certified professionals.

Now that we have discussed personnel, I would like to develop the administrative structure to a greater extent. The first organizational component that needs to be addressed deals with eligibility participation and discharge plan. The essential criteria for participation in the ADHC is the recommendation of a physician. This does not mean that a variety of other referral entities, such as discharge planners, case managers, or social workers from other organizations, cannot make the decision that ADHC is appropriate. What this criteria establishes is that the direct access to participation lies in the approval of the physician, who must state the principal and significant diagnoses, the prognoses and principal type of treatment, and the expected duration. The physician's order in the form of a written request to admit the person to ADHC program should also include overall therapeutic goals, needs for medications and special diets. Since few physicians at this point in time are apprised of the service components of ADHC, or how they function, the responsibility for briefing the physician usually rests with the referring agents, such as those mentioned above.

There should be a signed written agreement between the participant (or appropriate family representative) and the center. If necessary, appropriate documents can be obtained from an external funding source such as the Medicaid program. Very often the Medicaid program requires a prior authorization, which is a procedure that must take place at the time of recommendation by the physician.

Whether the ADHC is freestanding or institutional-based, there should be a geographical area from which it draws its participants and a set of standards that attempts to define the degree of frailty of applicants it hopes to serve. The ADHC will then be able to screen appropriately, and not find itself in a position whereby its population is either too sick or not sick enough for the existing staffing pattern.

Pre-Admission Assessment

Prior to admission the multi-disciplinary team should conduct an assessment that includes the primary diagnosis (i.e., staff physician's statement concerning the applicant), an assessment of the home environment and current living arrangements, the relationship with the informal support networks, and/or professional support systems. Assessment of the living arrangement should include an analysis of the heat, bathing, toileting and cooking facilities of the applicant's current home. Transportation, shopping and other environmental barriers should be incorporated into this initial assessment.

On admission, the multi-disciplinary team shall determine the medical, psychosocial and functional status of each patient, and develop an individualized plan of care, including goals, objectives, and specific services needed to meet the identified needs of the recipient. To assure that each member of the multi-disciplinary team "buys in," the entire team should sign a statement concurring with its mutual conclusions. The care plan should include, at least, the medical diagnosis, and medications and treatments, prescribed by the physician; the number of days attendance; the schedule; and the specific types, in units and frequencies, of individual services to be given. This assessment should also include the therapeutic goals and the duration of each of the individual treatments that will be rendered. Transportation, nutrition, specific activities, and the projected length of stay should all be a stated part of this care plan.

Discharge

Although there will be supportable reasons why certain people may require indefinite involvement in ADHC, the discharge plan should optimize the services offered in ADHC with the hope that the individual will be able to live without ADHC after an appropriate period of treatment. The discharge plan must include the support for continued involvement in the program should "graduation" not be possible. Since participation is voluntary, the discharge plan should be reviewed with the participant, as should the care plan. It is very important to elicit the positive support of the participant, because many a well-thought out care plan has been thwarted by the participant's own unwillingness to accept certain components of it. Since the admission documents, assessment plan and care plan must be implemented with the full co-operation of the participant, there should be careful attention given to a review with the participant, or with a guardian or conservator. It would be helpful in any case that the family or some other supportive person be involved in this review. The participant, although not obligated to become involved in the program, must sign an acknowledgement of acceptance into the program and intent to become involved.

Optional Services

We have described the basic services required in a good ADHC program. We should also be cognizant that certain other services are advisable if they can be obtained on a pro bono or contractual basis, such as podiatric care, dental screening and visual care. The ADHC program must plan, in their policies and procedures, to make arrangements for emergencies, should they occur, and should spend time organizing a transport service, which is the backbone of the success of their day care program.

HOME HEALTH SERVICES

Of all the health services in our continuum, caring for people at home has the longest historical precedent. In early America, physicians came to the home to treat their patients, and the family rendered the routine care needed the rest of the time. The hospital was viewed as a resource for people who could not afford home care. Home care programs per se, however, were developed in an effort to help the poor avoid the stigma attached to the necessity of coming to a hospital for care. In the 1800s home care services taught basic sanitation and methods for rendering care to the ill and their families. It wasn't until the latter part of the 1800s that home care organizations actually hired nurses to deliver direct service. Los Angeles County Health Department in 1898 was actually the first governmental health department that rendered direct nursing services to the sick poor in their homes. Many organizations, including insurance companies, developed home care programs that continued up to the late 1940s. In the early '40s hospitals began to provide home care for recently discharged patients. During this period, many agencies including hospitals, health associations, government and insurance companies offered home health services. Rather than explore the contemporary history of home health here, suffice it to say that the concept recently has received a tremendous boost as it relates to the needs of the homebound elderly.

In the early 1970s, when it became apparent that the institutional approach to caring for the elderly was not working properly, other elements of the continuum of care were sought as panaceas to this dilemma. The revitalization of the home care movement—as applied to the needs of the elderly population at risk of inappropriate institutionalization—became the leading "cause" of the advocates for the elderly. The following is a list of the traditional home health services commonly thought of in this context:

Homemaker Services (Sometimes Called Choreworker Services)

This person may do cooking, cleaning or shopping.

Home Health Aide

This person is trained to give hands-on services such as assistance in dressing, bathing, toileting, grooming. Often such training includes the ability to change dressings, give range of motions and assist in ambulation and basic exercise.

Visiting Nurse

A visiting nurse may render any service required of a registered nurse, including injections, medications, assessment and specialized treatment.

Social Service

This individual may hold a Master of Science of Social Work or may be a specially trained social service worker who can deal with conflicts, interpersonal and family relations, interpretation of benefit programs, and social service assessment in relation to the cultural and socialization needs of the individual.

Paramedical Specialists

Occupational therapists and physical therapists can render specific therapy modalities related to their professions. More important, though, is an emphasis on certain functional procedures which relate to the client's ability to perform the simple activities of daily living.

Medical Services

These are specific services that can only be rendered by a physician, and may include evaluation of drug regimen, direct medical treatments, or physical examinations.

It is quite plausible, and in fact, not uncommon, to have the senior service center and the senior outreach system as parts of the same organization. Later we will discuss models that exemplify this combination.

There is a clear natural interrelationship between these three community-oriented and noninstitutional service systems, which can be forged through appropriate administrative leadership—into a single effective working entity.

We have just described three major systems whose goal would be to maintain the frail elderly in their homes. We must now project a situation whereby certain percentage of those elderly will find their homes to be inadequate and require residence in a more protective environment.

Management Structure

We have briefly discussed the nature of the home health agency as it relates to the total system, and we will now review the administrative structure needed to deliver the services. The home health agency, as any other component of the continuum of care, is a highly structured service system that requires policies and procedures, documentation of various kinds, monitoring and re-evaluation. Because home health services are paid for through the federal Medicare program, the federal regulations that govern them usually set the framework for the organizational structure of the home health agency. Most states also require that home health agencies be licensed, even before they are approved for Medicare funding. And it is usually immaterial whether the home health agency is freestanding, institutional-based or part of a larger non-institutional organization, the requirements will be the same.

ADMINISTRATION

Although not required by federal regulations, I would recommend that the administrator of a home health agency have a certain minimum standard of executive management training, and have a degree, on a graduate level, in health management, health administration, or some comparable field. While it is totally appropriate to require that the administrator of a home health agency be a physician or a nurse, I strongly recommend that there be, at the least, these mandated academic requirements. Again, I take the position that the success of a home health agency will be due to its administration, and that administration will succeed primarily on the strength of its management competency and not necessarily on its clinical know-how. A properly trained manager will have marketing skills, fiscal skills, personnel management skills, and other administrative talents that can truly bring success to the organization. The clinical knowledge that person has (while being most valuable), simply is not as important as the leadership function.

The administrator of the home health agency will organize and direct all of the agency's activities and be the primary linkage to government, community and professional groups. The administrator will also be responsible for the development and implementation of policies and procedures that relate to direct services, employment of staff, budget, and all fiscal affairs. He or she will report directly to a governing body—an entity that assumes full legal authority and responsibility for the operation of the agency. If this is a non-profit home health agency, then it will be a non-profit governing board. If it is proprietary, then a corporate governing board will be designated. The full disclosure of the governing board must be written into the policies and procedures and is normally an important component of the application for certification. For a home health agency sponsored by a public entity, usually an elected governing body or a commission-appointed body represents the agency's higher authority.

Supervisory Leadership

The home health agency must have a supervising physician or supervising registered nurse. Under some circumstances this requirement could be covered by a qualified administrator. All of the therapeutic services rendered by the home health agency are under the direct supervision of this individual. Heavy emphasis, in therapeutic services, should be placed on the development of qualifications and the assignment of specific personnel to cases.

Basic Services

At the very minimum, part-time or intermittent skilled nursing and at least one other therapeutic modality, such as physical or occupational therapy, must be rendered by the home health agency. Most home health agencies offer two or more services, with at least one being under the auspices of the agency. Other sub-units of service can be contracted with another organization.

Patient Participation

There must be a realistic expectation that the elderly patient's needs can be met by the agency in the patient's home. Care can only follow after an assessment and written plan of treatment is developed, and then approved and monitored periodically by the primary physician. The plan of treatment includes a mental status evaluation and description of types of service and equipment required. It will be quite specific on the prognosis, the frequency of treatments, and should detail progress made with individual treatments as they relate to the total treatment plan. The plan will describe functional limitations of the patient and those activities that are permitted; also nutritional requirements, medications and treatments and any environmental requirements to insure safety, ambiance and good health. It is important to understand that the appropriateness of home care is a major polemic in the field of long term care. The controversy between institutional and non-institutional services and the appropriateness of either for a specific individual depends on a variety of factors which usually are made evident through the individual's assessment.

The basic economics compares the cost of keeping a person at home with the cost of staying in a nursing home. Through 1980 the cost of home care was relatively low (as we've discussed in other parts of this text). Since 1980, with the absorption of home health agencies by acute hospitals and the movement of proprietary home health agencies into the field, per unit cost, that is, per hour cost of service, has been driven up significantly. So, evaluating a person's need for home care on the basis of cost alone often may show that home care is disadvantageous, since it takes *less* than one hour of billed home care RN time to equal the total cost incurred in a 24-hour skilled nursing facility.

Since the economics at this point are so out of proportion with the services rendered, other values must be taken into account. Primary among these is the quality-of-life value of keeping the individual in his home environment. Opposing viewpoints discuss isolation and loneliness and the effect these factors have on regression; so these arguments too, must be taken into consideration. It is also worth noting, at this point, the absence of a sound emergency response system to home care programs.

Despite these apparent deficiencies of home care, though, its validity in a variety of circumstances has proven itself. Enter a new element of concern in the administration of home care. Just as difficulties are incurred in monitoring the performance of nurse assistants in institutions, there are equal difficulties in monitoring the performance of home health aides and other personnel who go into the privacy of a recipient's home. It would be wrong to assume that situations of patient abuse and neglect that, on occasion, are reported in the institutional sector, cannot possibly occur in the home care sector. It is the obligation of the administration of the home health agency tightly to monitor the conduct of the caregiver and the quality of services delivered. (A variety of techniques may be employed, but they definitely should include recipient feedback.) Allowing a careworker into the confines of a dependent adult's domicile offers opportunity for many abuses, and it is only through careful screening, training and monitoring of performance that defects in the home health care system can be controlled.

Nursing Service

The primary service rendered by the home health agency is supplied directly by or under the immediate supervision of a registered nurse. (In this case a licensed vocational nurse renders the service.) The registered nurse must be responsible for the initial evaluation and re-evaluation of the patient's nursing needs, and the initiation of the treatment plan and its periodic revision. The nurse must also define specialized skills and specific services, both preventive and rehabilitative, that will be applied to the treatment plan. He or she must maintain clinical notes, and co-ordinate a variety of other services needed to implement the total patient care plan. He or she has an integral role in communicating with family, other paraprofessionals and the physician, and has a teaching and supervisory role with other nursing personnel.

If there is a practical or licensed vocational nurse involved in the direct service, the performance of this individual is supervised by a registered nurse. He or she must be responsible for the same documentation, and recording, as required for the registered nurse. During the time that the licensed vocational nurse or practical nurse directly assists the physician or registered nurse, specifically-defined support duties will be assigned.

Rehabilitative Services

Occupational, physical and speech therapy are often rendered as part of the home health agency services. Each of these health specialties may offer qualified therapy assistants under immediate supervision by the professional. Each of these professionals must develop care plans, record progress notes, consultations, in-service programs, and the results and prognosis of their work.

Medical Social Services

Medical social services, when required as part of the care plan, are given either by a qualified social worker or by a qualified social worker assistant under the direct supervision of a social worker.

This form of professional support assists the physician and team members in understanding the social and emotional factors with which the care recipient must cope. The social service worker also participates in the development of the treatment plan, prepares clinical and progress notes, and documentation comparable to that of the other professionals rendering the service. The social service worker also works with the family and acts as a linkage to appropriate community resources, particularly when the recipient is about to be removed from the home care service program. The social service worker is also a vital link to other agencies and government departments.

Home Health Aides

Home health aides must be attitudinally appropriate to render personal and intimate care to the elderly person at home. They must be literate enough to conduct their component of the care plan as written. They must be able to document responses and progress as necessary. Aides are trained in methods that will allow the recipient maximum self-sufficiency with particular emphasis on assisting them in activities of daily living. Although the standards of the federal Medicaid program define the home health aide in broad terms, many organizations describe the individual who is responsible for housekeeping, cooking and shopping as a choreworker or homemaker. This differentiates the home health aide as one who actually renders hands-on care relating to toileting, dressing, bathing, grooming, ambulation training and certain treatments. Whether the home health aide has these "choreworker services" in their job description or not, it is advisable that this individual be trained to understand these particular needs and report them back to the agency.

For a variety of reasons, the home health aide assumes a level of great importance to the recipient. First of all, there is a probability that the actual number of hours of personal contact will be higher than for any of the other treatment modalities offered through the home health agency, and therefore a great deal more familiarity develops between the recipient and the home health aide.

Secondly, there seems to be a more intimate relationship developed in the services rendered by the home health aide than in those of the more technically trained professionals. Because of this, strong personal bonds often develop between the home health aide and the recipient, which sets the therapeutic role of the home health aide far above the specific services rendered. As we see with nurse aides in the institutional setting, the home health aide often becomes a confidante and a surrogate family member, and the nature of this interpersonal relation is often a strong supportive therapy in its own right.

System Relationships

Since the early 1980s, home care systems have changed organizationally due to their acquisition by the acute hospitals and the emergence of the proprietary home health agency. In point of fact the vast majority of growth in the home health agencies has occurred in these two sectors. Since 1983 there has been a clearer profitability factor than ever before, usually through the reimbursement mechanism for consumable supplies and for equipment. Since most of the profitability comes from these two items, any new governmental restriction on reimbursement would radically change profitability. The advantage to the acute hospital, in addition to potential profitability, is that home care allows a vertically integrated system of retaining patients within its own care network. Although the danger of self-serving referral and inappropriate retention of clients exists in this system, home care, as a service, will no doubt expand considerably.

There are problems of over-valuing home care. Recently it has been noted that home care programs may not be adequate for recently discharged elderlies who are much sicker due to the diagnostic-related grouping process. If the home care plan is not able to care totally for all of the patient's needs, then the element of risk of living alone exceeds the advantages of the system.

Another interesting relationship with the expansion of home care is the effect it has on the informal network. It is easy to see how some families or friends who are able to render care to a frail elderly person and who are under a great deal of stress in doing so as the person becomes incrementally sicker, are greatly relieved to have home care relieve them of the burden. While there is a great deal of dispute as to the shift or loss of the informal network support with the incursion of the home health care program, it could be that, to some extent, home health care service replaces informal caregiver service, and therefore, produces no net gain to the system that supports the elderly person.

The marketing of home health care programs has become one of the most sophisticated elements of long term care marketing. The competition for available paying patients is keen; while the numbers of people who are in need of home care, but who for some reason do not have a viable payment source, may be increasing. The fact that the profit orientation of the proprietary home care system exclusively addresses the paying population ignores the reality of an invisible population of elderly who truly need home care but to whom services can only be rendered by the public sector. It is therefore incumbent upon public sector sources, usually local health authorities, to be particularly tuned in to the elderly person who lacks existing government payment sources that allow him or her to receive home care. Concurrent with this line of thinking, we must recognize that if appropriate home care services are not rendered there is a high probability of either acute episodes causing re-admission to expensive acute care, or of inappropriate admission to skilled nursing facilities.

Home Care Financing

The vast majority of home care is financed through Medicare, Medicaid, Title 20 and the Older American Act. Small percentages are funded through personal insurance programs, HMOs and private resources. The American Hospital Association maintains a very valuable list of resources for finding homemaker and home health services. In 1979 GAO indicated that there was, in their words, "significant fraud and abuse" in certain homecare programs. Therefore, it is incumbent upon the administration and governing body of home health agencies to be meticulous in their documentation of fiscal affairs. The National Association of Home Health Agencies and the American Federation of Home Health Agencies are the "industry's voice" and are involved in public policy issues involving regulation and reimbursement at the federal level. Because home care is so labor-intensive, the federal government may limit costs by units of services. This plan may encourage the utilization of more units of service to cover basic expenses. This and other major economic issues face the administration of home health agencies. It is therefore imperative that the governance of the agency be more administratively sophisticated than ever before.

Senior Housing

Senior housing is one component of an array of discrete senior services for the frail elderly, for which there are many combinations of actual delivery. We will therefore define three basic prototypes which may be mixed or altered in ways that will become apparent as we further explore the continuum.

BASIC DESIGN

The basic senior housing is an apartment building with certain design features built in for the protection of the elderly resident. By this protection we mean safety enhancements that not only improve the security of the building, but remove typical hazards often encountered by elderly apartment dwellers. Many have options for communal dining (through contract) and a limited social/recreational program.

Senior housing should offer direct communication between the apartment and the manager's office, and, hopefully, some security at the front door. While there is no requirement that the manager need always be present, the intercom design should include some way to assure that the manager will know—even when not physically in his office—when his office has been buzzed. At present there are systems available that will allow for this level of communication. Another farsighted aspect of senior housing security will allow the elderly occupant to communicate quickly by radio or telephone to an emergency service network. Although not yet commonly utilized, various products now on the market allow this direct communication either from an apartment or from a beeper device worn by the elderly person directly to a nearby emergency coordinating unit. It is still rather uncommon to find.

DESIGN

Senior housing in its essential form has design features within the apartment such as elevated toilets, grab bars, and lowered "peepholes" at the front door. It also has cabinets in the kitchen that are usually lower, stoves and ovens designed for the particular needs of the elderly, and a trip-free floor design. While the emphasis in these design features is safety, there are a variety of environmental enhancements that can be made in terms of color, and decor that studies have shown will create a very positive environment.

One of the unfortunate circumstances of most senior housing is that there is limited space in the apartments. The transition from homes of their own to senior housing force the elderly to contract all of their worldly possessions to one closet, and the limited storage space in the basement of the building. This "contraction," as I call it, is a most difficult step for elderly people. For many it is the first real "cleaning out" of their possessions that they've had in years. Often items have to be given away, new bedroom sets purchased, and clothing inventories substantially reduced. There is rarely any assistance to the elderly in transition to senior housing. Therefore the trauma of this move is borne by them alone. One hopes such housing will show greater concern for this particular problem in the future, but because of the economics of building senior housing, living space is designed as minimal and concurrent storage space is usually quite limited.

All new senior housing must be designed for disabled people with doorways, ramps, elevators, and a variety of other features that will allow wheelchair access and egress. However, most existing senior housing does not have these features, and disabled people, even those in walkers, have limited mobility both within the building itself, and while exiting and entering.

Senior housing is designed in essence to enable residents to remain independent as long as possible in a safe, pleasant and efficient environment. It requires that they be able to cook their own meals, clean their own apartment and make use of a variety of services that the community offers them.

ASSISTED INDEPENDENT LIVING

As time goes on the elderly person may find himself in need of services. As stated earlier these services include so-called choreworker or homemaker services such as cleaning, shopping and cooking. Eventually a full range of support services may be needed for a resident. The concept of assisted independent living implies that on admission to the senior housing a network of services will be available and delivered on an as needed basis. The burden to produce these services falls on the management. Very often contractors such as home health agencies, homemakers' services, etc., will make arrangements with the management to provide these services to the occupants when needed. In our earlier discussions of the senior service center and the outreach service system, we outlined some of the most common of these offerings. What we are describing now, however, is an environment in which the elderly person may actually live and the process by which those services are supplied him on site.

The funding for assisted independent living can come through private pay for service, on arrangement, or through a government program such as Title 20 which pays for income support services for those eligible. To the best degree possible, the administration of the assisted dependent living project will be independent and not a contractor or provider of services. It will have no case management, or quality assurance responsibilities, and no other function than linking the resource with the party in need.

CONGREGATE HOUSING

This form of housing has a structured network of support services as part of the basic organization. The administrator—or manager—(a term more commonly used) of the facility is responsible both for the structuring of the financial relationship between the provider of service and the recipient, and for the management of these services. In some cases, the congregate housing organization itself pays for the services rendered and then collects from the resident; in others the administration arranges for a direct payor/payee relationship. While direct fee for service payment is the most common source of funding, Title 20, with its in-home support services section, and a few other governmental programs, will also fund congregate housing services.

Some congregate housing sites differ from basic senior housing in that they have centralized dining with mandatory participation. Other common services noted in congregate housing are social and recreational, housekeeping, home health aide services such as bathing and dressing, and home delivered meals.

Some congregate housing sites offer emergency medical and nursing services, paramedical therapy such as physical and occupational therapy, and social service consultation. Projects differ considerably depending on the funding sources. For example, those funded through government funding sources have a variety of regulations and operating conditions that are absent from privately funded projects. Government funded projects additionally have specific standards for the management of such facilities, and currently they may require managers to have certification through approved programs.

Problem Areas

Most states do not license independent living because it is viewed as a nonservice related entity. As more senior housing comes replete with services for the occupants, this viewpoint may change. Licensure of senior housing would almost certainly add a great many regulatory requirements to a very elemental operation. The licensure concept would automatically increase complication of running such a place and concurrently increase the cost of operations.

There are many examples, however, of independent living facilities that are almost indistinguishable from board and care or personal care units. When any senior housing development opens, there is a certain mean age of occupants. As time goes by, the mean age of this population increases, despite attrition of the older residents and the entry of younger seniors. Concurrent with this increase in mean age is a predictable increase of the service needs of that population. As the timeline or longevity of the project increases, the service needs of the population begin to increase almost logorhythmically, so that it is possible 10 years after the opening of a project to have an operation not dissimilar to a board and care facility.

Transfer Agreements

Because of this structural change in the population that lives in any given housing project, the management is faced with the need to discharge a person from that project to a setting appropriate to that individual's needs. If the independent housing project offers little or no services, the point at which those transfers are needed will be earlier in the timeline. If, on the other hand, it is a full-service congregate housing, transfers to a facility offering higher levels of care can be deferred for a while. In essence, independent living which offers no services, and congregate housing which offers many, will be housing populations with different ages and different levels of support service requirements.

One of the great difficulties facing housing sponsors and managers is defining the limitations of their facility to the applicant.

There must be a clear understanding on both the part of the applicant for senior housing and the management what the limitations are and what the requirements and standards are for discharging a resident to a higher service level situation.

Unfortunately, this situation is not at all clear in most organizations. The decision to move a person is traumatic to management and occupant alike. Very often there are inadequate community resources with which to handle the discharge and transition of this person; and if the facility does not have available support services in the community to help maintain the occupant's independence, then the discharge from senior housing becomes highly problematic.

The transfer problem is further complicated not only by the lack of resources in the community, but by the lack of a formal transfer agreement between the senior housing unit and the facility offering a higher degree of services. Without formal discharge agreements, there is no assurance that the person in need will have the opportunity to move to another facility. Very often this person may be forced to continue residing in the senior housing in extreme need of support services.

Sometimes, because of the lack of support services, a crisis will result which forces the discharge of the individual directly to a nursing home. This lack of transitional services often works to the disadvantage of the elderly person who suddenly finds himself in a situation where their presumed independence is lost immediately in a highly structured nursing home that has many more services than this person actually needs. Another major problem faced by management is minimal federal funding for plant maintenance and renovation. An abnormally high demand for services results in waiting lists and the interpersonal difficulties that arise when divergent people share adjacent housing.

ADMINISTRATION

In the field of housing administration, the top administrative person in any particular housing unit is called the manager. While there have been attempts for many years to certify all housing managers and to have a uniform training program applied throughout the country, we find, however, that the only certification program is for administrators of public housing. The Institute of Real Estate Management has certain training programs that qualify people as certified property managers or accredited resident managers. But, nevertheless, there is no continuity throughout the country, and therefore the field of housing management is yet to become a unified, stable profession. Many housing managers are what are called resident managers, in that they live in the facility.

The traditional housing manager's role consists of the following responsibility: (1) maintenance of standards as established by the ownership or governance; (2) monitoring operational expenses; (3) reporting of financial status; (4) contracting with local agencies for services and program; (5) direct supervision of the management personnel.

The housing manager will attempt to extend the limited program resources of the senior housing facility by encouraging volunteer activities amongst the residents and developing some social and recreational activity program. The good housing manager knows the individuals in the facility on a personal level, and is able to address personal needs and problems as they arise. While the housing manager is usually not trained in social work or related services, they are pressed into dealing with a myriad of personal problems. Most housing managers have resources to deal with particularly difficult cases through social service agencies or specialized health consultants.

A good housing manager will know the capabilities and limitations of each of his residents and will have a list of personal supports that can be brought to any problem that may arise with a specific resident. The name of the doctor, spiritual member, or family member would form the backbone of such a support team. At all times the supports should be directed towards helping the resident maintain independent functioning and self-sufficiency. The housing manager must have a superb ability to communicate and utilize his communications skills to a maximum.

The most successful approach for social programming is the development of the residents' council or resident organization, with a variety of subcommittees, such as welcoming committee, social program committee, buildings and grounds committee, etc. These residents' committees can be designed so that they themselves handle complaints, and to some degree, monitor the various operations of the housing facility. The existence of a residents' organization allows easy flow of suggestions and problem-solving. It also puts a self-governance concept into play that in itself through peer pressure and peer counseling deals with many problems that in other circumstances must be dealt with by professional staff.

Housing managers must factor in ongoing training and inservice training for the few staff that usually work as part of the management team. Many housing managers take courses in gerontology or social services, and others assume, of course, where they ultimately achieve a graduate level degree. There is no mandate for a bachelor degree, but as the field progresses, most positions will be occupied by college educated, professionally-oriented individuals.

Some of the basic functions that must take place under the housing manager include the following: (1) managing, application, and admission process; (2) payment of bills, collection of rent, and related fiscal function; (3) budget preparation; (4) accounting and cost control; (5) assuring the routine cleaning and maintenance of physical plant; (6) the development of job descriptions, the recruitment, training and supervision of all staff; (7) the ongoing decorating and refurbishing of units; (8) the inspection and assurance that fire and safety standards are being met; (9) addressing problems relating to the termination of tenancy, including eviction and transfer to other services or level of care.

Besides these basic administrative functions are certain services that are appropriate for housing for the elderly, such as security and related issues, the installation of adaptive devices where needed, counseling the residents, referral of the resident to more appropriate services such as residential care or congregate housing, if appropriate, and the linkage of the resident with outside help and social services appropriate to that person's needs.

Residential Care

In some areas, residential care is called board and care, in others it is called boarding home for the aged, and in some geographic areas it may be called adult residential care home. Regardless of the specific local title, we are describing a non-health facility which offers basic services that are fairly consistent throughout the country. In our discussion of the history of long term care, we noted that with the inception of the social security laws, we found the old boarding homes expanding to meet the needs of the elderly during the latter part of the 1930s. The social security component which helped fund this expansion of what were at the time called "rest homes," was the O.A.S.I., or Old Age Survivor's Insurance. The "rest home" has become a generic name for any residence which houses an elderly person. Lay people often confuse or use the term "rest home" when describing a skilled nursing facility. It is better, however, to use this lay term to describe a residential care home or a board and care home. In the last few years the term health-related facility has entered the lexicon in long term care. A health-related facility, for all intents and purposes, is a board and care facility with the availability of personal care services. A health-related facility (HRF) is often contiguous with, or a component of, a multi-service facility. As such, it draws upon the health technology of the skilled nursing or acute units. Residential care homes which meet the needs of the more frail elderly population often find that there is only a semantic difference between rendering residential care and intermediate or skilled nursing care. For example, the in-house population, over a period of time, may age substantially and, for whatever reason, the most frail cannot be discharged to a medical facility such as an intermediate care or skilled nursing facility. In these situations, the "homes" themselves are responsible for rendering whatever services are needed. If one looked at these facilities, one would see a high service residential care, with many walkers and wheelchairs, and intense services which relate to the activities of daily living. In these facilities, which are often called personal care units, one will see incontinence and many people who fluctuate at certain times during the week into a category that would be more clearly labelled intermediate care or skilled nursing. The existence of this service-intensive component of the residential care field has led to new definitions of programs such as "health-related facility," that actually do address the gap between the "rest home" and the nursing facility.

Most states have no licensing or certification for the administrators of these facilities and there is a consistent pattern of minimizing the standards for this particular position, when in reality we find, once again, that the administrator's education, experience, and overall competency is the primary determinant of the quality of services rendered within the facility. True, most of the facilities are quite small, and this argues against having an "overly trained" individual, if for no other reason than the economics of hiring such a person. Most standards for the administrative position require someone of good character with appropriate experience in dealing with the institutional needs of the elderly. Usually these standards are minimal, and rarely is there ever the requirement for an advanced education of any kind.

What one finds is that most of the small residential care facilities are run on a family basis. Usually the owner will have a converted residence or other small edifice that has been converted to accommodate the residential care needs of the occupants. Very often the administrator/owner is a nurse or licensed vocational nurse. It is uncommon to find a person with an appropriate bachelor's degree or the management capability to address fiscal and planning needs. The academic and experiential base to address the humane psychosocial milieu required for the benefit of the resident is often lacking.

ADMINISTRATIVE ORGANIZATION

The residential care needs of an elderly individual are not well defined, nor is there a discrete body of knowledge for that level of service. We find that as in hospice, as noted before, the qualifications and standards set for the administrator tend to be vague and ambiguous. As students of health administration, we find it difficult to view a non-health human service organization with little formal structure and no mandatory academic and experiential requirements relating specifically to the needs of the elderly population in the facility. My own inclination is to require a graduate degree in some form of human service. This allows the individual not only a full range of academic knowledge of the elderly, but requires enough management training to allow that individual to function properly in the administrative role. Most of the facilities are relatively small, the vast majority being six or fewer beds. Even the larger facilities in this genre of human service organization are only between ten and fifteen units. In the larger retirement centers, continuing care facilities, and multi-level non-profit organizations, we do, of course find residential care service homes that are larger and do require (and usually have) someone with more extensive academic training and management in human service delivery. But in essence the field of residential care homes is one of relatively small units run by individuals who create, at best, a familial atmosphere about the home and, because of this, are able to do an adequate job for the resident.

While most of these facilities are licensed by the state, they do not require the administrator to be either licensed or certified, nor to go through any testing process. There are a few states which require specific academic training or on-going continuing education, as is required of most other professional administrative positions in human service. Administrator and licensee may be the same person, the only requirement being that the administrator have sufficient freedom from other responsibilities to permit adequate attention to the management and administration of the facility. Most states require that they have the knowledge for providing care and supervision appropriate to the residents, as well as knowledge of the variety of laws, rules and regulations required to operate the facility. They must demonstrate the ability to manage the fiscal records and have the capability to supervise and direct the work of others. They must demonstrate good character and have a reputation for personal integrity. The states which do require some advanced education and/or training usually base this requirement on the size of the facility; for example, they may require that the administrator of a facility licensed from sixteen to forty-nine beds would have one level of required college education, while an administrator of fifty or more beds should have, perhaps, a bachelor's degree, with allowance for experiential equivalence. Some of the states which have been more attentive to this particular field are requiring continuing education in the area of serving the elderly, or in administration.

I have proposed for some time that administrators of residential care, regardless of size, be licensed or certified, and undergo rigorous state testing and monitoring. In the end analysis everything flows across the administrator's desk. Though the licensee or governing body is ultimately responsible for operation of the facility, it does not have direct responsibility for the implementation of regulations. We must assume, regardless of what external mandates exist, that everything—funnelled as it is across the administrator's desk—is interpreted and implemented on the basis of that individual's overall capability. The best laid plans of governmental public policy will succeed or fail on the basis of administrative skill, and while this theory can be applied to all the service delivery organizations, it is especially obvious in this particular sector due to the minimalist approach to academic and experiential requirements. Licensing and/or certification at least would put the administrator in a more visible (and therefore more controllable) position. If there *were* problems with the organization the administrator then would face the potential loss of license or certification to do business. But even more important than this, licensure and certification would start to develop the administration of residential care facilities into a profession in its own right. This form of movement indeed would upgrade not only the profession of administering this kind of facility, but the ultimate quality of services delivered. In my opinion, this would be a very significant factor in improving the all-around quality of care and service rendered in residential care facilities.

One of the main responsibilities that the administrator has in residential care is to implement governmental rules and regulations and establish internal operational policies and procedures, in order to allow delivery of specific services. The internal program, which includes a structured array of services, both required and otherwise, collectively brings to the residents the opportunity to live a complete life. Yet most residential care facilities lack extensive resources, and essentially operate from revenues received from Social Security Income (SSI) or minimal private resources. In other words, few residential care facilities have the outside community support which allows them to offer much more than the basic amenities of living. In the not-for-profit sector, there is an answer of sorts in organizations whose constituencies, through donating money or offering direct services, are able to expand their resource base and offer a much higher quality of life to residents. Unfortunately these organizations are in the minority.

Regardless of the size of the facility, administrators should develop an administrative plan which clearly defines policies and procedures. Lines of responsibility, workloads, job descriptions, and the duties of any supervisory personnel should be spelled out.

As in other comparable administrative positions, the administrator must be responsible for recruiting, employing, and training qualified staff, and by the same token take responsibility for terminating employees who do not perform adequately. The administrator must assure that the facility provides services that relate appropriately to the physical and mental needs of the residents. A pre-admission appraisal or assessment will be the guiding document that will determine what these needs are. It is important that this assessment also determine whether the facility is actually able to offer the type or level of services needed. Often those needs which cannot be met by the residential care home can be met by community programs; neighborhood, or governmental programs, or the service of proprietary service agencies. As we have seen from our discussion of the continuum of care, there are many non-institutional support services in communities. Senior centers and outreach service systems are but two. It is very common for non-institutional services to support people in residential care settings. Transportation to senior centers for recreational programming, health-oriented support clinics, and so on, are just a few of the services which could be made available through astute administration to the residents of the residential care facility.

The administrator also must be responsible for the personnel records and payroll records. These resident records, which should include the demographics of the resident, a health history, and the pre-admission assessment or appraisal. The administrator is responsible for assuring that there is adequate staff to perform office work, cooking, housecleaning, laundry, and maintenance of building and grounds. There must be adequate service personnel to address the daily living needs and the social and recreational needs of the population, as required in the organization's list of basic services. All employees must be given some form of training related to the job assigned. For example, food service workers must have training in the principles of good nutrition, food preparation, food storage, and menu planning. Housekeepers must be trained and re-trained in sanitation principles and housekeeping techniques. Direct service personnel must be trained in the skill and knowledge required for direct resident care, as prescribed in the basic services. All must be trained in safety, fire prevention, and possible emergency situations. Therefore, a major administrative duty is the design of on-the-job training programs, skilled training, and the development of continuing education. As it may be very difficult actually to implement these programs, it is imperative that the administrator be aware of the community resources that can be utilized for this form of training.

BASIC SERVICES

Basic services rendered by the residential care facility should seek to encourage the independence and self-direction of all persons within the facility. Beyond this, it is the responsibility of administration to provide a safe and healthy living environment with three nutritionally well-balanced meals, snacks when necessary, and other modified diets which can be accommodated by the kitchen. It is important that the nutritional capabilities of the facility be made known to the practitioner and resident prior to admission. There should be observation of the resident's physical and mental conditions, as well as the ability to assist in toileting, bathing, dressing, and eating as necessary. It is also required that the facility assist the resident in taking prescription medicine and arrange for his or her health needs, which may include setting up transportation to a physician or health clinic. A basic service that is required in all residential care facilities is to have some form of acceptable planned activity program which encourages socialization and offers recreational activities that enhance the environment for the residents. The physical structure of the residential care facility should encourage socialization and be adequate to allow the resident space to move about unencumbered (including space to allow assistive devices such as wheelchairs or walkers). It is very important that the facility take the responsibility of observing the resident to determine if there are unmet needs which might require additional services unavailable in a residential care facility. The facility also must arrange resident's medical and dental services and must assist residents with self-administered medications or treatments.

The planned activities which are most appropriate deal with socialization, daily living skills, and recreational and leisure time activities. To some extent, physical activities (such as games or sports or exercises) may be appropriate, depending on the abilities of the residents. Consistent with our psycho-social model, creative and educational programs are equally important to the growth and development of the elderly person. A major challenge for the administrator is to be able to utilize community resources such as church, senior centers, and neighborhood organizations in addressing these educational and creative needs. Attendance at a place of worship is often an excellent component of the services rendered by the residential care facility.

INTEGRATED RESIDENTIAL SERVICES

We have been discussing those freestanding residential care facilities which have an administrative paradigm of their own. Let us now examine a residential care unit in a multi-service facility such as often seen in life-care or continuing-care organizations or multi-level not-for-profit homes for the aged. Regulations and licensure for these components of larger, more complex organizations are normally the same, but find that the administration is much more complicated. Under normal circumstances, there is one administrator for the entire complex, with possibly an assistant administrator who specializes in the residential care facility. The administration of a residential care unit within this multi-care organization has characteristics of the administration of the other subcomponents. For example, the need to integrate services is foremost in that people move from one level of service to another. The movement of the resident from one level of services to another in a multi-level organization is often very traumatic, to the resident, and very difficult from an administrative standpoint. The residential care unit is an integrated department in a total delivery system, and as such, plays an entirely different role than a free-standing unit.

First of all, the multi-level service organization which we have described normally has responsibilities to residents for continuing, or life-care, and therefore must be able to supply services which do not meet the norm. For example, if a person living in the residential care unit needs nursing services, those resources are brought in; or else the occupant is brought for a short time into the nursing unit. By the same token, if the people in the independent living unit need residential support services, these services may be brought to the independent living unit, or else residents of the unit may go, for a short period of time, to the residential care unit. The sharing of resources in this matter gives the resident of the multi-service organization a tremendous spectrum of potential services with which to meet many more contingencies than would exist in a unit which must rely on a relatively fixed staff to render services, i.e., the free-standing unit. Multi-level facilities, whose primary services is residential care, normally have smaller skilled nursing units, sometimes called infirmaries, and may even have a small acute hospital unit. Although the basic regulations apply to this unit, because it is part of a larger organization there may be additional regulations which make it conform to guidelines for continuing life-care facilities. Therefore, there will be different admission procedures, economic implications, and management strategies for the development of this programming within the facility. Relationships between residents of different levels within the facility are all factors that must be taken into account in running the total organization. Because of this additional complexity, and the need to know a variety of somewhat different care level delivery systems, the administration we have just described is much more difficult. In most cases it requires graduate education, not only to deal with fiscal management, but to deal with the complexities of different dimensions of care and their integration into a single successful working entity. As a matter of fact, many large residential care facilities, whether they be free-standing or integrated within a multi-level organization, find it a necessity to develop different levels of residential care. The most labor-intensive or service-intensive type of residential care is called personal care. Very often personal care is more of a phenomenon than a designed level of care. It defines the situation within a closed system that has a population whose mean age increases with time. As the age of the population of the residential care facility increases, so does the average level of medical acuity. There comes a time, not too long after certain residential facilities begin, that they have higher levels of frail elderly who border on needing intermediate or skilled nursing care.

This grey area between residential care and skilled nursing care, often is accommodated by the facility in what are called personal care units, which add incremental amounts of nursing services to what is considered a residential care unit. Very often, in a personal care unit, you will find wheelchairs, walkers, and people whose debility may in other circumstances be considered nursing cases. The residential care unit often is without discharge options due to limitations of space within its own skilled nursing facility, or else a variety of barriers prevent discharge of the resident to an outside skilled nursing facility. Consequently, the facility is pressed to offer these additional nursing services in a residential care unit to prevent the anticipated transfer shock and to keep patients in the friendly and familiar environment of their own residential area. Personal care units are closely watched by state regulatory agencies to assure that the appropriate services are being rendered and that transfers out of that service are made successfully when truly mandated by the resident's condition. The administrator must develop a mechanism to monitor the fluctuating medical profiles of people in the personal care unit much more intensely than in any of the residential care levels. By virtue of being the most frail, these residents are the most volatile in terms of short term periodic needs for more intensive observation and nursing assistance. As we know, this age group demonstrates amplitudinal changes in medical acuity anyway, and this particular component of the residential care population is even more prone to have short term periods when nursing care is needed. During the winter months, this frail population is much more subject to debilitating pneumonias and other serious seasonal conditions than are other members of the residential care unit. These characteristics of the population in personal care resemble, to a marked degree, those of the intermediate care population. Sometimes a personal care unit is called a health-related facility and has the opportunity to be licensed as such. The health-related facility designation allows for a clearer definition of a residential care setting which has the need for periodic short term health-oriented services. In a health-related facility, these services are available to a greater extent than in a personal care unit, but in essence we are addressing a very similar population. The health-related facility must pay greater attention to documentation of services rendered the resident than would normally be required in a residential care setting. What is most important is that the administrator must appreciate the limitations of the health-related facility's capabilities, so that residents are not cared for in an environment which really cannot fully meet their needs. This requires constant monitoring on the part of all caregivers in the health related facility to assure that appropriate services are being rendered to residents. A "red flag" can be waved when those service levels are exceeded by the resident's own needs. As we have discussed with senior housing or independent living, it is very important that a discharge plan be drawn up and monitored very carefully, particularly for the personal care or health-related facility clientele. It is quite possible that this discharge plan may be activated with very little notice. The discharge plan (or transfer plan, as it is called in many cases), must be agreed upon at admission, and must contain in it the obligations of both the management of the residential care unit and the resident or the resident's conservator. It must define the criteria determining the point at which the resident will be discharged to a higher level of service. These criteria should be consistent for the population as a whole and not be directed towards any one particular individual. The administration must be closely involved with the progress of any single resident in order to be certain that these criteria, when met, do activate the discharge program, and that the discharge site is available and can assist in making the transition as smooth as possible. Very often, residents will agree to this form of transfer or discharge understanding, but because they have become accommodated to the residential care unit, they need a great deal of encouragement to get them to comply with the original understanding. It is very difficult to move a person who has been in a comfortable residential care setting to a more medically intensive environment without incurring transfer trauma. Although the existence of transfer trauma has been challenged, this author feels very strongly that it is a mentally debilitating assault on a resident to be moved without appropriate prior counseling, proper transition during the move, and supportive, familiar human contact at the discharge site. A variety of studies have been done to alleviate and reduce the extent of trauma, using social service counseling techniques.

One form of residential care which has not been discussed is that which allows the resident to stay in place in place in a single living accommodation, and brings a variety of services to that one location. This means that as the person ages and becomes more debilitated, services are brought to the person's abode rather than moving the person to more intensive service locations. Hence, services are rendered on a very flexible basis, and the person is able to remain in residential care, although receiving nursing services either from an external source or from another unit within the multi-service organization. There are some organizations which believe this to be the most appropriate delivery of services, even to the point of retaining a person who is very near the acute hospital phase. While this kind of service *can* be rendered and managed properly, we must realize that it is quite expensive and fails to maximize the benefits of good organization that come from a specialized unit.

It is my opinion that there will be many permutations of the residential care concept as expansion of the institutional component continues. Ideally, the residential care unit will be an integrated component of the long term care continuum, which avails itself fully of all the non-institutional services we have described thus far.

Hospice

No discussion of the long term care system would be complete without inclusion of hospice, and while the newly-defined hospice system in this country does not have stereotypical administrative structures, we can at least describe its function and services and extrapolate to some degree the type of leadership and organizational structure which would be needed.

Current hospice concept evolved from the concern of many people that the traditional health care system was unable appropriately to care for the person with a life-threatening illness. Some even took the position that because of the societal emphasis on cure and recovery there was actually hostility toward the dying patient. This set the stage for covert abandonment of appropriate care where there was a negative prognosis. The long term care system, which concentrates on frail elderly, has more exposure to the terminally ill by virtue of its clientele. But even in these cases concern has been expressed as to whether the terminally ill were being cared for properly.

The best way to define a hospice is by describing some of the principal services rendered in a hospice concept. First of all, the patient and his or her family are factored into the care process. An interdisciplinary team is assembled which will respond not only to the medical, but to the spiritual and psychosocial needs of the patient and family.

A major emphasis will be placed on symptomatic treatment and pain control and great consideration given to followup with the family in terms of dealing with grief and emotional suffering. Hospice, for all intents and purposes, need not be an actual place, but rather a concept or philosophy that seeks to "restore dignity" to the dying person, and add, at terminus, a sense of uplifting fulfillment. The goal of hospice is to improve the quality of life for the person who otherwise may be stripped of dignity and die in loneliness and pain.

The first time that hospice principles were applied in this country was in 1899 at the Calvary Hospital in The Bronx, New York, but the primary example of hospice care was St. Christopher's Hospice in England, which opened in 1967. Since this time, according to the National Hospice Organization, several hundred hospices have been opened throughout the U.S.A. Recent federal legislation has offered some minimal form of economic support through the Medicare program. A hospice program may be either institutionally-based or in the form of home care, and some projects are combinations of both. Included in a comprehensive hospice care program would be: (1) physician service; (2) skilled nursing care; (3) home health care; (4) physical, speech, and occupational therapies; (5) pain relief treatment; (6) emotional support services; and (7) spiritual support. A hospice may have a contractual relationship with another agency to perform services that they are unable to render and therefore a referral network is often established. This allows the recipient to receive all of these benefits as part of one integrated program.

While the standards of administrative and organizational design (beyond the specific Medicare regulations) are still in the developmental stage, in our current system, it is totally appropriate for a person—either a physician, nurse, or social worker—with graduate credentials and experience in dealing with the dying patient to be the administrator. Since management determines whether or not an organization will be viable, the administrator should also have adequate management education, hopefully in the form of a graduate degree. Because of the humanistic approach taken by most hospices, the organizations often minimize "structural" management processes that are common throughout the health field. The result, though, is that many hospices may not be adequately managed. As this system evolves, the requirements for more sophisticated managerial control will become obvious. At this stage, however, the clinical experience and professional education of the staff and leadership are still the primary criteria for employment. Volunteers are a crucial factor to the success of the hospice program, and in many cases families who have benefitted from hospice become ongoing volunteers to assist in maintaining the program's level of activity.

While Medicare is the primary source of funding for hospice care, Medicaid, Title XX, special grants, governmental contracts, and private payment are also important sources, as are organizational donations and hospital revenues that in some cases underwrite hospital-based hospice units.

One of the more unique aspects of hospice care is the high rate of burnout of employees and volunteers connected with the program.

Normal stress is exacerbated by the intense involvement caregivers have, and the inevitable frustrations that develop when a great effort goes into the care of a dying patient. Most hospice programs have special mechanisms for dealing with conflict, hostility, and depression, which are often the manifestations of this stress. Better training orientation and selection are necessary for stable hospice operation, and special support programs designed to deal with the needs of staff and volunteers in this stressful environment need also be developed.

The organization of hospice from a management standpoint is so ambiguous that federal regulations do not define the administrative role beyond mandating the existence of a governing body, which assumes full legal responsibility for all aspects of the hospice operation. This body then must appoint someone who is responsible for the day-to-day operation of the hospice. The hospice itself must provide or arrange for all of the services which are described in the written agreement with the recipient. It must also assure that there is continuity of care, whether at home as an outpatient or as an inpatient. Regardless of the locus of the service, the hospice with which the patient contracts has the mandate to professionally manage all services.

The plan of care is developed by the multi-disciplinary team, and includes assessment, implementation, monitoring, and re-evaluation. Other components of the hospice program are an ongoing quality assurance process, continued in-service training of employees, and the utilization of an acceptable, informed consent form which specifies not only the type of care and services the program will render, but guarantees not to discontinue or diminish care, should there be some problem with the recipient's ability to pay. To comply with the guidelines, the hospice must document certain minimum standards for volunteers activity, guarantee availability of clergy, and maintain specifically designed clinical records to ensure that appropriate ongoing utilization review and quality assurance can be maintained for licensure. The multi-disciplinary team must include at least a physician, a registered nurse, a social worker, and pastoral care or similar counselling. Other members of this team are related to various support therapies. Volunteers may also be included.

Federal regulations require strict management of staff time, maintenance of core services, and clearly define the professional standards of the participants in the multi-disciplinary team. The criteria for supply usage, services rendered by therapeutic support personnel, and specific guidelines for in-patient home care hospice service indicate that what once was rather an amorphous collection of poorly defined services rendered by well-intentioned people has now become a relatively structured professional component of the health system. While there may not be the specific managerial structure common to most other services in the continuum, it appears that the atypical administrative design of the hospice meets the needs of the recipient, and obviously complies with the federal regulations which currently govern hospice programs.

INTERNAL MANAGEMENT, SKILLED NURSING FACILITY

The skilled nursing facility is the most complex entity within the continuum. It is also the component of the continuum where the most professional and public attention is focused. As I've mentioned in previous chapters, the organizational structure of a skilled nursing facility is derivative of the acute hospital. As we explore the internal management of the skilled nursing facility, we will continually relate various aspects of the management to other issues we have discussed in this book, i.e., the continuum of care, historical relevance of any particular aspect of internal management, and resident-oriented decision making.

When we trace the historical development of the long term care system, we see that, from early on, the relationship of skilled nursing facility to acute hospital was always that of the poor cousin. The first regulations for the skilled nursing facility were watered down acute hospital regulations. The standards for it set on both federal and state levels were, in many ways, replications of the medical model. So, for most intents and purposes, the internal management of the skilled nursing facility is the same as that found in the acute hospital, rather than its own, unique model.

Only upon examining the impact of limited resources in the contact of a lower level technology can we begin to understand some of the problems in internal management and see some of the real reasons for misunderstandings over the end result in nursing home service delivery. Skilled nursing facilities are almost always smaller, in budgetary and personnel terms, than their acute counterparts. But it is not size (as closer scrutiny of internal management practice will reveal) but the mini-acute mentality prevailing in a non-acute facility that is more likely to be a source of administrative problems and misunderstanding. What follows is a more functional description of departmental operations which would relate to regulatory requirements. We will be outlining, in a somewhat linear and traditional fashion, the departmental set up of a typical facility; and then discussing the possibilities for integrating of these departmental functions. The concept of a managed environment can then be laid over this breakdown to describe the actual operation—the internal management—of the nursing home. The challenge to the skilled administrator of a nursing home is to bridge the gap between the traditional pyramidal structure of top down management, and the total environmental approach of the managed environment. In fact, these two approaches to the structure of the skilled nursing facility are not necessarily contradictory; they can be, rather, fused together in the service of our primary goal: a patient-oriented management system.

The first step in describing internal management is to utilize the basic services that are required by state and federal laws, and from these basic services form the elemental nursing home organization. We have already discussed the external management component and we will assume that the administrator is at the top of the organizational chart. We will only occasionally relate internal management to the governance of the facility.

Once this organizational structure is schematicized we will then progressively add facets to the structure that, in most cases, are not required by law. We will have an opportunity to describe those facilities that offer services above and beyond minimal legal requirements. One advantage we have in discussing this topic is that there is a surprising level of homogeneity in the services rendered between skilled nursing facilities. Since federal laws standardize all basic services we have, at least, a nucleus of services that one will find from one end of the country to the other. Even with the surprising degree of standardization that has taken place in the last few years, the system is not totally static. We will also explore those standards that allow individuals to be cared for in a skilled nursing facility, recognizing that there are fluctuations in the application of these standards throughout the system.

BASIC ORGANIZATIONAL DESIGN

The basic required services for an SNF are physician services, nursing services: dietetic, pharmaceutical, activity and administrative services. The administrative services would include fiscal, housekeeping, and buildings and maintenance. All of the services of the nursing home must be broken down into those that are "line," part of the authority structure, and those that are "staff" or consultative.

Before we go further and analyze the authoritarian responsibility vested in the leaders of each of these key departments, I think we should acknowledge that the administrator of a nursing home is very close to front-line operations, and does not have the luxury of having organizational barriers between him and the action. You will find in most cases, that administrators spend a considerable amount of time "in the halls" and cannot divorce themselves in true "executive" fashion from the dynamics of care being rendered in his facility. The buffers that are common to hospital administrators are not available to the nursing home administrator, and without those elements of protection, he is exposed to the raw emotional content of his facility. By this I mean that he is constantly available to both resident and family, and therefore must share in the varied conflicts that those groups produce. We will expore the administrative role in greater depth, but let us first describe the basic organization in terms of traditional definitions of functions.

First of all, ideally no more than five to seven individuals should report directly to the administrator. There have been many organizational analyses of what is called span of control. Because the administrator is directly involved in many aspects of management that do not relate directly to the functioning of his subordinates (i.e., family and community issues), the smaller the span of control is, the more effective the administrator can be. We are describing, at this initial stage of investigation, a traditional, organizational chart with the apparent investiture of responsibility to the department heads and the delegation of comparable authority to allow them to carry out these responsibilities. The perception created by the shape of this organizational chart (implying a "top down" administration) can be modified by the style of administration that is practiced. Certainly the "top down" approach may be appropriate when an organization is going through a process of change. As this period of change increases, a different administrative style will probably be indicated—one that will allow for long range stability and some degree of balance. In mature organizations, a variety of collective approaches to management including group decision making, and derivative planning and program development activities, are not uncommon. It is the unwise administrator who assumes that his organization does not have the capability for grass roots input in management. The result of this attitude often results in a rigid, disinterested organization that sooner or later runs into management-oriented, resident care problems.

Nursing Service

The nursing service is the primary service in the long term care facility; all other activities in the nursing home interface and support it. By taking this position—simply a description of the reality of nursing home operation—we open an administrative can of worms. By defining one service as a primary (more important service), we concurrently define other services as less important. This process of defining a hierarchy in very small working units creates many operational problems, and directs us to see a possible solution where the perception of hierarchy is reversed and some element of equality is designed into the organization.

Rather than discussing the Director of Nurses first (the more traditional approach), I am going to deal instead with the unit of personnel that is most significantly involved with the well-being of the residents, and their quality of life: that is the nurse aide or nursing assistant. This is to say that the quality of life in a nursing home is no better or worse than the quality of services supplied by these particular individuals. It is appropriate, I feel, to discuss them first and then move up the hierarchy to describe the leadership needed to make this unit successful. The administrator who delegates care on the basis of a resume, interview, and traditional hiring approach puts all his eggs in one basket when it comes to employing a competent Director of Nursing. He presupposes that this Director of Nursing understands the dynamics of direct care delivery. This is an important point. Many an administrator has lost not only the first battle through this misunderstanding—but the entire war. The traditional way of hiring a DON *must* be augmented by a real working knowledge of patient care dynamics on the administrator's part as well as on the part of the Director of Nurses.

The nursing assistant gives direct bedside care and has more hours of contact with the residents in a skilled nursing facility than any other member of the staff. It is an intimate and personal form of contact, neither distant nor academic. It is the kind of contact that makes a good day or a bad day for residents, the kind of contact that must be finely tuned in order to be successful. Fortunately, the intimate bedside care we are discussing is not fraught with a high level of technical substance, but relates to the high feeling level that must exist in the delivery of this service. If this feeling level between the nurse assistant and the resident is not high and positive, the technical accomplishments of the nurse assistant are irrelevant. They will have little effect on the quality of life of the resident. In recent years, nurses aides, or nurse assistants, have required certification. This has been one of the most significant factors in the improvement of patient care in SNFs since the inception of this field of care. The certification process has required both the knowledge of nursing techniques and some psychosocial information. The nurse assistant now understands the psychosocial dynamics that exist in the aging process (between the resident, herself and the family) better than ever before.

Throughout the country the majority of nurse assistants, at least in urban areas, come from third world neighborhoods and work in facilities primarily populated by white, middle class people. In rural areas this is not so, and you find that the nurse assistant is drawn from whatever socioethnic culture exists in that particular rural area. Recognizing though that the majority come from different strata of our society than those that are cared for defines potential sources of conflict between caregiver and care receiver. The nurse assistant performs a list of basic bedside nursing services day in and day out. The work is repetitious, physically demanding, and (certainly as normal patient regressive cycles take place), very emotionally draining.

From an administrator's viewpoint, the primary concern with the nursing department will be delivering adequate nurse hours of service to meet the needs of the resident and be in compliance with the regulations that govern your facility. Do not be deluded into thinking you are running a quality facility just because you are above state standards. These standards, by and large, are minimums, and cannot be viewed in any ethical way as models of peak operation (although, unfortunately, a great number of administrators view them as such).

An additional standard of measurement of nursing performance—the fundamental standard—is the nurse aide or nurse assistant ratio. That is the number of patients one nurse aide is assigned to on the day shift. Some people have alleged that nurse hour ratios have little validity because of the wide variability of acuity in any patient population. It is my view that it is these critics who view standards as ceilings, and not floors. Many years ago I concluded that minimal standards must be accepted to prevent the "floor" from being even lower than it is. Each day the nurse assistant must do a laundry list of such services. When there are too many patients per assistant, some of these services will simply not get done. Even worse is that when demands are excessive on the nurses assistants, the human component of service—far more important than the technological component—is the first to go. Residents are dressed and addressed abruptly, or not spoken to at all, rushed in and out of the bath and shower, and hurried when eating. Sometimes the food tray is removed prematurely because of the workload, an action deeply upsetting to a resident who has made this meal the focus of the day.

Some people maintain that the measure of productivity of nurse aides is the number of units served they can deliver in any particular hour. For example, the nurse aide who can bathe six people in an hour is more productive and therefore more desirable than a person who can bathe four people in an hour. This is a highly debatable viewpoint. The idea that you can quantify direct human service in this manner, and relate that to quality of life, is mostly untrue. Few of the readers of this text would appreciate being rushed in and out of a shower, especially if it was one of two showers a week assigned to you, with no interaction, no touching, no calming words—handled, so to speak—like a sack of grain.

The following ratio should be adequate to prevent this sort of low-grade treatment: in the average nursing home, ranges of 1 to 6 up to 1 to 7 seem to be adequate in dealing with the basic needs of the "typical" patient. Ratios of 1 to 8 and above are excessive and cannot produce quality work. One to 5 ratios are ideal, and are found in most private facilities.

The attempt to set staffing or nurse hour ratios is complicated. Detractors claim that in any one given patient population there's such significant variability that the establishment of standards is pointless. If one were to make the statement that 7 to 1 is an acceptable ratio, it could be pointed out that there are certain residents who require significantly lighter care, and that this level of care (7:1) is excessive, and in point of fact, wasteful. One could also point out that certain facilities would have very heavy care patients or even the fact that cyclically there is a significant change in the patient population that says in essence one day a 1 to 7 may appear adequate, and the next day it may not be adequate because of the admission of many heavy care cases. Certainly the point that is being addressed, i.e., the amplitudinal change in the medical profile in any nursing home is true. It is also true that admissions of heavy care or significantly light care patients alter the day-to-day job required of the nurse aid or assistant population. What I am suggesting, however, is that these variations require adjustments, but that basic mean standards be established as minimum standards. It certainly couldn't be argued, that a 1:7 ratio would be able to deal with severely handicapped patients that needed extra care or that the addition of staff would not be welcomed. On the other hand, we've seen situations where the typical nursing home population is served by a single nurse aide caring for 9 or 10 or 11, as is the case in our current system, and this must be considered inadequate.

Nurse aide ratios and nurse hour standards are very meaningful when an administrator must deal with the fiscal management of the facility. You will find that the nursing department is the largest personnel component in your budget. It would, therefore, make sense that tightly controlling this personnel unit would relate directly to the fiscal viability and profitability, if this is a profit making nursing home. Poor care, however, will have its own effect on profitability. Few private pay cases will be referred, and fines, citations and litigation are always on the horizon.

MIDDLE MANAGEMENT

In a small unit such as an SNF, it is unusual to view the charge nurse as middle management; yet, if one were to examine the staffing patterns of countless nursing homes throughout the country, the charge nurse (registered nurse or a licensed vocational (practical) nurse), is the frontline supervisor and the individual through whom hospital policy and state and federal regulations must be filtered. Since we are working our way up the organizational hierarchy, we must describe these middle managers in terms of their real responsibilities. It should be noted that in most states registered nurses are not required "around the clock" and practical nurses or licensed vocational nurses may be charge nurses in most smaller facilities on the evening and night shifts. This means that there is a definite possibility in the smaller facility that the entire managerial control will be in the hands of a licensed vocational nurse, who has had no more than 12 to 18 months education in techniques of this profession. Noticeably absent from the curricula in this professional education is training in the function for which they are truly held accountable: management and supervision. While I call them middle management there's no doubt that their function is primarily supervisory. The lack of a significant management component in the curricula for licensed vocational nurses or in the state test, certainly is a tremendous weakness in the system. The charge nurse, regardless of what license she works under, has direct supervisory responsibility over a unit of nurse aides and must therefore assure the DON that the assignments given the nurse aides have been taken care of. The licensed nurse lacking any training in supervision and being selected for her job primarily on the merits of her license, is in a very difficult spot. Her own work performance will be judged on her basis as a supervisor and unit manager, and not necessarily on her technical knowledge. If one were to break up the average day of the middle manager, one would find an imbalance between the supervisory function and the technical/management component of any particular job. The balance, unfortunately, would favor the paperwork component of required documentation for medications, treatments, etc., in proportion to time spent on their supervisory function.

In determining the number of licensed personnel needed to act in this pivotal role, we do not have tidy ratios to guide us. Federal regulations require several staffing patterns, which will be noted in the regulations. Again, though, we find that these staffing requirements are minimalist and are designed essentially to allow the licensed person enough time to comply with the many and varied regulations that they are responsible for compliance. Unfortunately, we get to the issue that compliance in terms of federal and state regulatory bodies normally means the documentation of proof of rendering of service. The services are specifically spelled out in the regulations, and this process of documentation for compliance (and the rendering of certain services specifically related to their licensure) does not include the very important time elements needed to supervise the nursing assistants. If one were to review the job assignments of most nursing supervisors, there would be a noticeable lack of time allocated to supervisory functions. While the new direction of governmental surveys will be directed to "outcome" evaluation through patient assessment, the lack of adequate supervisory time will still be critical.

DIRECTOR OF NURSES

We now are going to discuss the most important person in a nursing home, the Director of Nurses. It is with some trepidation, that I use the term "most important" because it immediately puts all others in a subordinate position, but it is my belief that the DON makes the patient care system run. The DON in an SNF is required to be a registered nurse, ideally with appropriate service in long term care and an education that confirms that she understands the needs of the elderly and disabled patient. In the early stages of development of the nursing home system, the vast majority of DONs were those that were near retirement or nurses with acute hospital backgrounds who were new entries in the field. It was rare to find a DON who had chosen long term care as a field of endeavor, or who had been specifically trained for this field. Lately we have seen evidence that more younger nurses with at least a modest background in geriatrics are entering the field. It should be noted, however, that although the curricula for undergraduate nurses is being expanded in many places throughout the country, it is primarily being directed towards the involvement of the registered nurse in the acute hospital population of elderly. Hopefully, as the needs of the elderly population are translated into curricula, there will emerge a greater emphasis on the social component of care. Certainly the training of those individuals who become DONs in SNFs is an important issue in health training today. If one were to analyze the actual responsibilities and day-to-day activities of the DON, you would find that her need for geriatric nursing per se (i.e., dealing directly with the pathology or medical model) is relatively limited. Her primary function is that of a manager, a supervisor, a coordinator, a public relations specialist, and a problem solver. There have been many administrators that have hired a nurse and enthused over her rare background in geriatric training, only to find that those characteristics most needed were nowhere in her experience. This won't become manifest until many operational problems develop that are directly related to the lack of managerial capabilities. Eventually, if the point is made after a couple of years, the training of the geriatric nurse will include heavy emphasis on management and supervision, and a concurrent parallel training in the psychosocial needs in the elderly in a variety of settings, including the institutional.

In addition to being responsible for managing the nursing staff, the DON must also coordinate the activities of virtually all of the paramedical specialists. While it may be the responsibility of the administrator to recruit and contract these paramedical services, it is the responsibility of the DON to integrate them to the care plan.

COORDINATING FUNCTION OF THE DON

All of the paramedical specialists that function in a nursing home function through the DON. Their performance should be evaluated by her, and their progress monitored by her.

This woman, were she working in the acute hospital system, would make anywhere from 30 to 50% more salary for the same level of responsibility. The family interaction functions of the DON are a reality of the game. It is very difficult to get through the day without some family related problem. The DON also may be the main contact person for community in that certain care questions may best be answered by her. While the community and public contacts may be the primary responsibility of the administrator, most family contacts are in the domain of the DON. So here we are describing a situation where the DON not only manages the nursing staff in compliance with all state and federal regulations, but also coordinates the involvement of a large number of medical specialists, links up with the medical director, and the medical community, and deals with discharges and the concomitant problems that develop. She is also the primary source for most administrative communication with families.

To some extent, based on her capability, the DON's responsibility can be reduced. For example, it may be that another individual on the staff is best suited for communicating with the family, perhaps it is the activity worker, or maybe even the administrator. There are many combinations.

Another interesting aspect of the DON's expanded responsibility, especially as they relate to public relations, is that a high percentage of the visits from families come in the evening or on weekends. Normally the DON is not at the facility during these times, and therefore the responsibility for public relations falls on the charge nurse during these shifts. Communication with the public, particularly family, is often shifted to the nurse assistant in at these times. This particular communication link has been one of the most unfortunate aspects in the delivery of nursing home care. Not only does the nurse assistant not have adequate knowledge to communicate to the family the medical picture, very often the nurse assistant does not have the communications skills to relay more than the most elemental description of the patient being discussed. What happens because of this communication gap and misperception by the family of the nurse assistant's responsibility for conditions in the facility, is that a significant conflict develops between the two. There is every reason to believe that a substantial number of complaints about nursing home care stems not from negligent care, but is a derivative of the conflict that develops between a nurse assistant and a family person. Consequently, those administrators that are able to train their nurse assistants in the art of communicating with families will radically decrease the number of complaints and patient care problems reported by families.

ECONOMIC RAMIFICATIONS OF STAFFING AND TRAINING

Although the ramifications of proper staffing and training apply to most departments in an SNF, it can be said that many problems are directly related to the nursing service in this regard. The most important benefit is, of course, the proper treatment of the resident in the long term care facility, the recognition of his total needs and the enhancement of the persons quality of life. Proper staffing will create a positive public image, but, even more importantly, will reduce the possibility of a negative image, and repeated lawsuits and conflicts with community and family groups. Most regulatory violations that cause fines and other legal difficulties stem from poor patient care that can be directly attributed to improper staffing, training and supervision. Expensive turnover, reduced use of sicktime and overtime, and little or no ability to attract private pay patients are some of the expected results of improper staffing. The administrator that uses internal staffing patterns as a way to improve his profits or reduce a deficit will soon find out that the indirect expenses incurred with poor staffing will easily outweigh savings from light staffing patterns.

Dietary Department

DIETARY SERVICE

The primary purpose of the Dietary Service Department is to provide for proper resident nutrition. This euphemistic definition sometimes flies in the face of regulations, traditional medical practice, and the reality of the low budget food service. In order for an administrator to have a properly run dietary service, he must know certain unique characteristics of food service in the nursing home. Food service rarely reaches its potential in most facilities, because of the heavy emphasis placed on following the regulations (which must be done). Following the regulations means that your food service is primarily medically-oriented, and flows from the doctor in the form of a diet order. This diet order is recorded both in the resident's chart and in some form of record in the food service department. In most cases you will find that the medical training of the physician and his experience in the acute hospital will lead him to request an array of diets not normally within the nursing home capability to produce. Most nursing homes, therefore, have a limited variety of specialized diets that they can, with a high degree of assurance, produce for the resident. This "diet manual" should be made available to the physician so that he knows from the beginning of his relationship with the SNF what is available for his own residents.

The ability to produce a wider range of diets enhances both the medical capability and resident satisfaction in the nursing home. Unfortunately, it puts a greater burden on the dietary department to assure quality in those traditional types of diets that are most frequently prescribed—diets that must continue to be produced on a daily basis.

Nutrition as taught in medical schools to physicians and to the dietetic profession utilizes data and information derived from studies of primarily middle-aged and younger-aged people. The specific needs of the elderly population (as would be expected) have not been given a great deal of consideration. Thus we get a pattern of dietary orders from the physician that attempt the same therapeutic processes normally applied to patients in acute care; for example, food delivered to the resident's bedside, i.e., salt-free, bland, low roughage and low fat diets are standard fare for elderly residents. While all of this seems appropriate, there is a significant amount of debate as to whether this degree of rigidity is truly necessary. Why must we apply acute hospital standards when serving the needs of elderly people who have, as one of life's few and primary pleasures, the need for familiar dietary food patterns often going back three or four decades? What about those who thrive only on ethnic food? We see here the conflict between acute hospital technology and the reality of long term living. We see also, in response to this dilemma, a new pattern of food service emerging that is not therapeutic, per se, but rather a part of the total quality-of-life pattern that we are trying to develop in the skilled nursing facility.

Let me extend this a little bit further. Most nursing home residents pace their day by their food service. Because the meal time is the period of the day that residents eagerly anticipate and plan for, it takes on a grander significance than what may be the relatively unimportant therapeutic effect of the food itself. Depending on which study you believe, residents aged 82—the average age in nursing homes, have lost a substantial portion of the tastebuds on their tongue, and therefore have a reduced ability to taste. Visualize, therefore, an 80-year-old resident receiving at his or her bedside a restrictive diet that lacks certain condiments and that doesn't relate in any way to the food pattern which that person has existed on for decades. The food services is in technical compliance with the regulations, but the resident is sadly deprived of the much-needed "gestalt" of the dining experience.

Visualize an alternative approach: a situation where the resident is brought to this food in a social environment of communal dining, where he has an assigned place that he can count on, and an assigned tablemate that affords him verbal or nonverbal opportunities for communication. The room in which the communal dining takes place is attractively designed, and the people who serve the food have been trained in interpersonal communications, so that they are able to further enhance the dining experience. As an added nicety, a more liberal or laissez-faire attitude is taken in the preparation of his special diet, so that certain condiments are added to it, compensating, however slightly, for his lost taste sensation. The plate and/or tray are thoughtfully arranged and balanced in terms of color, and some attention is given, if possible, to the person's ethnic, racial or national food preferences. Can you imagine the psychological difference?

What I am describing may sound to some like a dream, but in fact, many high-quality nursing homes *do* have communal dining rooms, flexible menus, non-restrictive diets, and make sincere efforts to comply with personalized food needs. The dietary enhancement of the quality of life is a most significant factor in the care provided by that facility. It is the administrator's responsibility to design his system to maximize the dining experience. He must not be deluded by assumptions of increased costs and fears of conflict with the medical community. If one were to evaluate the cost differential between the service I describe and the service that is commonly provided in nursing homes, one would find a difference of only pennies in cost per meal, per day. The positive atmosphere portrayed by this kind of dining experience has measurable impacts upon staff, residents and families alike. It takes little imagination to quantify, not only physically but in terms of dollars and cents, these apparently intangible enhancements. When the morale of both residents and staff is high, waste is reduced, and costs are effectively controlled.

STAFFING

The day-to-day operation of the dietary department in an SNF is run by a food service manager or director of food service. This individual is usually trained to the level of a "step two" dietary assistant. The training of this newly emerging position (and concurrent new emerging profession) varies considerably throughout the country, but emphasizes elements of nutrition, purchasing, sanitation, supervision, production, and food service delivery. As might be expected, most of these curricula do not adequately address significant areas such as supervision, conflict resolution, basic administration, problem solving and planning, which unfortunately usually occupy the majority of time of the food service manager. If the administrator is aware that the basic training is deficient in these key areas, he will make an effort to offer this key staff person opportunities to improve capabilities in those strategic areas. Running a kitchen on a day-to-day basis is a tough job. Resources, in terms of manpower, are usually stretched very thin, and the accountability, in terms of cost control and production control, can be quite restrictive. A great deal of responsibility is placed on this relatively untrained individual, who often gives yeoman service for a very moderately salaried position.

Individuals that are supervised by the food service manager are an array of cooks, cooks' helpers, kitchen helpers, dishwashers and kitchen janitorial helpers. There are different hierarchies in the cook establishment, which may normally be divided into first, second and third cook; first, second, third night cook; early cook; and so on. Although the name of this position varies, there is usually one top person, who has the most experience, that will be called the head cook. A normal 99 bed nursing home, for example, will have two cooks on duty during the day shift: one coming in quite early to assure that breakfast is on; and the other coming in slightly before noon to take the responsibility for the evening meal. The overlapping shifts provide enough manpower for the largest meal of the day, which is usually the noon meal. Most food service staff receive training that emphasizes sanitation, production and personal hygiene. Some elements of nutrition may be incorporated. As part of the enlightened administrator's approach to training, however, the entire food service staff should be brought into the quality care concept, and should be made to feel part of a total program to enhance the life of the residents. It is very easy, because the kitchen is somewhat removed from direct resident involvement, for the dietary service to feel remote and uninvolved. This disaffiliation causes more problems than any other single characteristic of the dietary service. If the group feels uninvolved and unimportant, their work will be careless, disinterested, and hazardous. If they are disaffiliated from the quality of life of the resident, hygiene, sanitation and aesthetic needs will become matters of indifference to them. If, on the other hand, they are brought into the resident care process, and made to recognize the importance of their work, they will be much more concerned with these important issues. It will be that much easier to get hygienic and artistically-prepared plates and trays from the dietary staff and positive interpersonal communication.

Contact between the dietary worker and the resident in a communal dining situation is most important. The dietary worker should be encouraged to consider himself part of the therapy team whenever he makes contact with the resident in the dining room. Once again, the importance of bringing all of the food service people into the therapeutic process cannot be overlooked.

At last we come to the dietitian, the best-trained (academically and experientially) member of the dietary team. In the vast majority of nursing homes, the dietitian acts as a consultant, and is only on the premises a few hours a month. Since the dietitian brings the highest level of professional input into the system, this consulting service must be relied upon to overview the therapeutic component diets, to assure proper menu planning and to assist, monitor and evaluate overall performance. This function must include written surveys and reports that are presented to the food service manager and administrator. While there are certain specific components of the regulations that can only be performed by a dietitian, the quality control function is far and above the most important. It is hoped that you will have a dietitian that has some knowledge of the needs of the elderly institutional population. While this training is rare, it would be good advice to encourage the dietary consultant to seek appropriate training on the nutritional needs of the elderly, and make it a required part of the contract of service.

RULES AND REGULATIONS

The governmental regulations for running a dietary department indicate a heavy emphasis on sanitation. On inspections, most of the time spent by the regulatory people will be on the evaluation of sanitary control. It is, therefore, wise to make sure that these issues are covered thoroughly before you address the real needs of your residents, which is the creation of a total positive dining experience.

Dietitian

Each licensed skilled nursing facility must have a professional dietitian either in a staff or consulting capacity. The number of hours of the service may vary, according to the size of the nursing home. Dietitians may have varied educational backgrounds, but should at the very least, be a member of the American Dietetic Association, whose standards should guarantee a consultant with credible academician and experiential background.

The role of the dietitian in a skilled nursing facility has been difficult to define and varies quite a bit due to variations of their particular background and to the capabilities of the food service supervisor. As the long term care field evolved, it became quite apparent that there were very few professional dietitians who had significant knowledge of the needs of the elderly or long term care resident. Most of them, in these earlier days, learned on the job and were able to modify through trial and error the somewhat parochial education they had received. This education was primarily oriented towards acute hospitals. In fact, most of the critical training required of dietitians is in acute hospitals.

This process of training dietitians in acute hospital organization and administration had initially proven to be a barrier to appropriate functioning of the dietitian in the long term care facility, because the LTC facilities operate on such different economic and nutritional parameters. After years of evolution, however, dietitians who now serve the nursing home field have had the opportunity for some long term care academic and experiential training. It is important, when hiring the dietitian, however, to ascertain exactly what the individual's contact has been with long term care. You will very often find a presumption on the part of the dietitian that they know the elderly's needs, only to find that they have expanded upon their acute hospital base of knowledge. Most acute hospital trained people have done this, and assumed that what was learned in the acute setting could be transferred to long term care. It is my opinion that the operational knowledge to serve the needs of the elderly in a long term care setting cannot be extrapolated from acute care without appropriate training and experience.

The dietitian's role in a skilled nursing facility is not normally managerially oriented. His or her time is usually spent in the more technical aspects of the nutritional component of the food service. These are, at the very minimum: assessment to evaluation of the residents' needs; and planning of the nutritional program. It is important that these responsibilities be extended to monitoring the success of this plan and any subsequent changes that may be needed.

As required by regulations, the dietary assessments and food service plans must be modified periodically, at least quarterly. The more effective dietitians—recognizing variability in the health profile of the elderly resident—are able to modify the plans to an even shorter cycle.

The dietitian is also integral to the development of the menu plan. She can assist the food service supervisor in making the necessary modifications to any particular day's menu and supply specifications on food, quantities to be cooked, and the technical alterations needed with new menus for special diets. Another very important role that the dietitian can play is that of an educator—there are many occasions when the nursing home health team evaluates the changing health needs of the residents and, at those times, nutritional advice and instruction will be needed.

Menu Planning

Not only can the dietitian become involved in assisting with traditional forms of menu planning, but it is a good use of the dietitian's time to take part in organizing the resident input into the menu planning process. A menu planning committee composed of residents, family and volunteers, is a most effective way to allow resident input in menu changes. These meetings also permit direct communication from the dietitian to the residents regarding technical questions involving the food service.

Very often these menu planning committees act as a release valve for the residents' frustrations with institutional living, which very often focus on the food service. The selective inclusion of family and volunteers also creates an atmosphere of involvement and flexibility that can reduce the severity of conflict areas that arise between resident and institution, and between family and institution. If handled properly, menu planning committees can even be fun for all parties concerned and produce constructive changes in the food service plan.

The administrator must be aware of certain inherent problems in the relationship with the consulting professional. The primary contact that the dietitian will have in the facility is with the food service director, and this relationship must be defined very carefully. Under normal circumstances the food service director is a top management person in the department and must report directly to administration. What this implies is that the consulting dietitian is not the consulting supervisor of the food service manager, but the professional consultant for those areas in which she is professionally competent. This point is being raised because the administrator must make a decision as to who is being held responsible for the operation of the dietary department. It is my recommendation that the food service manager have this responsibility, and that the overview and monitoring of quality control be placed as the responsibility of the consulting dietitian.

Another area that is often clouded is the relationship between the Medical Director and the dietitian. In many cases since the role of the Medical Director is not that of a clinical practitioner, the traditional line of responsibility that the dietitian has in an acute situation does not exist here. Certainly the dietitian has a responsibility to talk to the primary physician, who is in charge of the resident's health and who should be apprised of those circumstances that relate to nutrition. This, therefore, is another role of the dietitian, that of consulting with the primary physician.

The administrator should set up periodic meetings with the dietitian to not only monitor the dietitian's performance, but to keep in touch with her evaluation of the performance of the entire dietary service.

Food Service Supervisor

The food service supervisor is a full time position that is administratively responsible for the total dietary service. As mentioned before, this individual usually meets standards set by state law, and may be considered a dietetic technician by the standards set by the American Dietetic Association. Very often the food service supervisor has worked his/her way up through the ranks and has an intimate knowledge of a kitchen operation. Another characteristic of the food service supervisor is that she is close enough to resident care to have a very good knowledge of the individual likes and dislikes of the different residents; and when the opportunity arises may be able to accommodate these individual needs. While the educational background of the food service supervisor is significantly different than the registered dietitian who you will have as your consultant, the supervisor is in essence responsible to the administrator for the nutritional well being of the resident population. The most important characteristic this individual must have is skill in supervision, and as a component of the supervisory responsibility, the ability to recruit, select, train, and retain staff for the food service operation. Finding the right individual to perform these functions is a most difficult task, because most of the people who work in food service are untrained, and to some extent, noted for their transient habits.

The ability of the food supervisor to produce the planned menus on time and in an appropriate fashion is the basic measure of his or her supervisory ability. This person is also responsible for purchasing of food and consumable supplies, sanitation, and record keeping, which includes diet prescriptions as required by regulation. This person will also be a primary focus during licensing and certification inspections, and most administrators find that they rely heavily on the food supervisor for the success of these visits.

Because the supervisor is so "operationally oriented" it is important that he/she have the capability of working effectively with other departments, primarily the nursing department. Lines of communicat ion should be clear. Procedures for changing individual resident menus, for routing diet orders from physicians, and for alterations in any particular resident's meal must be worked through smoothly, or they will become points of conflict between departments.

Again, I will stress the importance of allowing the resident access to the food delivery system. The most viable way is through development of the menu planning committee, which brings in resident input, as well as family or volunteer participation. As noted before, the menu planning committee can recognize individual needs, act as a clearinghouse for resident problems with food service, and can reduce substantially the traditional conflict area between the institution and those it serves. It must be recognized that in addition to the three meals a day, the skilled nursing facility must be prepared to offer a mid-morning, afternoon and bedtime snack opportunity. Each of these components of the total meal service should be taken up for discussion by the menu planning committee.

POLICIES AND PROCEDURES

For each department in the skilled nursing facility a set of policies and procedures must be developed. While these policies and procedures use as their starting point specific regulations that relate to departmental operations, each facility is somewhat different, and therefore, policies and procedures must be customized.

One component of these policies and procedures is the diet manual, which lists a specific number of special diets that will be produced by the kitchen. Since most nursing home kitchens limit the number of special diets to 8 or 10, you will find the need to communicate with and educate the primary physicians who have residents in the skilled nursing facility. Most of them are used to the large array of special diets offered by the acute hospital and will very often prescribe diets that are not consistent with the nursing home diet manual. This educational process can be most easily accomplished by sending the primary physician a copy of the manual with an explanatory note. Most will be able to modify their diet orders to match the production capability of the skilled nursing facility kitchen.

The diet manual should, as we stated before, be reviewed annually by the resident care committee of the skilled nursing facility for the required annual update. The departmental procedures will include requirements for equipment maintenance, food storage, diet order recording, meal assessment, resident meal plans, etc.

Staffing

The staffing of the dietary service will vary depending upon the type of meal service selected. Differences in staffing, will hinge upon the presence or absence of communal dining room service. Communal dining, on the other hand, requires more manpower, because individuals are served at a table. Because tablemates often have conflicts and people have difficulty in comporting themselves in a dining room, additional management will be needed in communal dining rooms. Nonetheless, it is the best form of food service that a facility can offer. As we have discussed before, food service is not merely the intake of a nutritional product, but a total experience: the ambiance of the room, the companionship of a tablemate, and the aesthetics of a tastefully presented meal create a high point in the otherwise monotonous day of an institutionalized person.

When a person designs his day around socialized dining, the ability of a skilled nursing facility to create these heightened and eagerly-anticipated experiences during the day is a major contribution towards the enhancement of the quality of life of the resident.

Food service personnel who directly serve and interact with the residents must be specially trained for this interaction, because their relationship should be supportive to the elderly person in the dining room. In this way, the food service worker becomes a direct member of the health care team of the facility, must be treated in that fashion, and must know his/her importance to the total success of the institution's service.

Staff Meals

Traditionally people who work in the kitchen receive their meals gratis. Most other staff should be fed in the facility, and the most economical way to do this is to develop a cafeteria style meal service. Staff should be afforded the opportunity of purchasing low cost, nutritious food for their own meal breaks.

To be consistent with our resident centered administrative concept, the food service should be designed around the needs of the resident, and not around the needs of the health establishment. This may sound like a difficult thing to implement, but most physicians will recognize that it is more important to serve the personal wishes and desires of an 85-year-old person than to stick to a technical, medically appropriate nutritional regimen that may not offer appropriate life satisfaction. This potential conflict with traditional medical practice can often be avoided with proper communication with the primary physician, who, when given the opportunity, will agree with this quality of life issue.

Housekeeping Department

The Housekeeping Department is usually managed by an individual called the Head Housekeeper or Director of Housekeeping, normally a person who has worked his or her way up through the ranks—hopefully one who has a high school diploma. In some cases, this person may be called the Executive Housekeeper, which indicates some form of certification, or even an academic degree—such as an Associate of Arts degree. Sometimes you will find the Head or Executive Housekeeper in a nursing home has been trained in an acute hospital setting. This is one of the transfers of technological training that really benefits the skilled nursing facility because, normally, the in-service training rendered in an acute hospital for this type of person is usually appropriate to the needs of the skilled nursing facility. The basic techniques of mopping, dusting and cleaning learned in an acute hospital often form the basis for on-the-job training of other housekeeping staff, which consists of housekeepers (sometimes called maids) and porters. It is encouraged that traditional ways of allocating jobs between male and female personnel in this department be avoided and that both male and female have equal access to different types of assignments (which would mean that females might be mopping halls or lifting, and males might be cleaning rooms and toilets). This particular department thrives on the existence of a well thought through set of policies and procedures that are rigorously followed, and with ongoing, in-service training that reinforces these practices and procedures over and over again. This is one particular department where rigidity of assignment, scheduling and supervision are often the most successful tools to good department morale and long-term success. The greater the level of discipline and higher morale, the more successful this department will be, they will keep the place clean, utilizing materials appropriately and have successful inter-departmental relationships, while performing a unique role in the patient-interactive environment.

The housekeeper is one of the few people who, with a great deal of consistency, enters the immediate environment of a patient and as such becomes a surrogate daughter or son to the patient. It is very common in this concept of managed environment that the housekeeper—who is in the immediate vicinity of the patient daily—is told things that are never heard by the higher level professional staff. It is common for the patient to take the housekeeper into his or her confidence and for the housekeeper to bring the patient into his or her immediate family life. They will let the patient know about the trials and tribulations of a son/daughter/husband or friend, or take a similar approach to sharing family or private life with the isolated patient. This relationship between the housekeeper and the patient must be explored thoroughly. Once understood, it is easy to see why the housekeeper should be on one of the multi-disciplinary teams that develop patient programs and analyze patient care plans. For these reasons you will find that some of the best information about a patient comes from the housekeeper rather than nurse, paramedical, or medical practitioner. This invaluable input often is excluded by artibrarily downgrading the value of this potentially unique relationship with the resident.

Besides basic cleaning, the Housekeeping Department is usually responsible for most of the moving of furniture and boxes and equipment. It utilizes the infection control technology from the acute hospital. Most nursing homes have policies that require that the head housekeeper be on the infection control committee and it is to the advantage of the nursing home to make sure that the housekeeper has every opportunity to train and maintain current knowledge of infection control techniques as well as supervision, materials management and other aspects that relate to their job.

The primary inter-departmental relationship that the housekeeping department has is with nursing and the admission personnel. It is very important that beds become available as soon as they are vacated and that the admission department notifies the Housekeeping department when admissions and discharges are to take place. Good communication between Housekeeping and Nursing Services is very important, and lack of it causes traditional conflicts between these two departments. For instance, turf battles might arise over the nursing department's responsibility for cleaning up patient "accidents" (resident incontinence). Another point of conflict might revolve around who makes the beds and is responsible for cleaning the beds and bedside cabinets. In some facilities, this is the assigned task of the nurse aide, in other instances, the housekeeper.

The housekeeper, as well as the nurse aide, often form the patient's family in the surrogate fashion I have described. By virtue of the relationship the housekeeper forms with the patient, the Housekeeper may also become a *confidante* to the family and friend of the patient. Whenever this happens, a very healthy linkage is formed to the outside world.

The most common problem in this department is supervision. Normally, people who work their way up the ranks, or fit into the leadership category in this department, do so because of their tenacity and their knowledge of the actual workings of the job. The administrator must be very attentive to supervisory abilities of the housekeeper because much weight is placed on the cleanliness of the facility—above and beyond the regulatory requirements. What I am referring to is the reality that many people still judge a skilled nursing facility by how clean it looks, totally disregarding all other aspects. I have seen occasions where even professionals in the field judge the successful operation of a skilled nursing facility by how clean and shiny the floors are. Though this may be an archaic way to judge the quality of nursing care, it still exists in the minds of many people. The administration must realize that this organizational component has a function—again—above and beyond meeting regulatory requirements. It is vital that the administrator, or another member of the administration, make frequent documented rounds of the physical plant to assure that policies and procedures in this department are being carried out. Communication between Nursing and Housekeeping takes on another form when we realize that most of the requests for services outside of the normal work schedule come from nursing. Lines of communication have to be thought through and agreed upon in advance, otherwise a direct approach between a nursing aide and a housekeeper results in conflict.

The most successful line of communication is between a Nursing supervisor and a Housekeeping supervisor who then passes the request down the department hierarchy. Most housekeeping departments (as all other departments in a nursing home) are very thinly staffed; therefore, if a housekeeper does not show up, there must be contingency plans either to float or to arrange for one of the other housekeepers to take on an expanded job. It is a serious management error to have no pre-arranged fallback position for the part of the work force that does not show up for work—for whatever reason. Once Housekeeping services begin to operate effectively, they sometimes disappear from the administrator's view, due to the administrator's own pressing workload. It is important to realize that review and monitoring of the efficacy of the Housekeeping Department should be a routinely planned activity of the administrator, regardless of work pressures. If other needs are consistently seen as more pressing, this department may well let its performance deteriorate. Planned, periodic technical evaluations, of the use of chemicals and materials; quality, in-service training; analysis of workload distribution and absenteeism rates, are all good management tools.

LAUNDRY DEPARTMENT

In most facilities, the Laundry Department is the responsibility of the Head (or executive) Housekeeper. It has, as its most obvious responsibility, the processing, distribution and storage of linen and garments. Sometimes, under the Laundry Department, an individual is assigned to maintain clothing inventory. This position cost is money well spent. Lost, destroyed, or unclean clothing is a most unsatisfactory situation in a nursing home. Besides the obvious impact poor clothing management has on the patient, it creates serious problems with families and other interested parties. Too many times, we allow clothing management to become an unassigned task—one that "just sort of" happens or "just sort of" doesn't.

The laundry person, again, is someone who usually works up through the ranks and hopefully has had acute hospital or commercial laundry training. There are associations of laundry managers and a great deal of technological information can be obtained through these industry associations—standard, in-service training, wash formulas (the blend of the chemicals used in the washing machine) maintenance training, and so on. One of the nice things about the laundry department, is that its productivity is relatively easy to measure. Most standards of laundry measurement are often produced in pounds per day, pounds per patient day, and cost per pound. The use of these standards will enable you to compare the success of your laundry with commercial laundries, as well as with other facilities. In larger facilities, the economics of laundry production are improved by having more automated equipment and lower staff costs. Usually, the function of mending linen and clothing is assigned to the laundry department—i.e., to one of the staff that has these skills. Finally, the laundry is an important part of the infection control program and must have specific policies and procedures to deal with infectious linen. Clothing management should therefore be defined and incorporated into the job description of one or two individuals.

Conflicts also arise over the distribution of the linen. For example: whose responsibility is it to take the linen from the laundry to the wards? Most of the time, it is the laundry room's responsibility but, in some cases, the nursing service must go to the laundry and pick up the daily linen requirements. There are many standards for laundry operation. One of the standards is the set number of changes per bed per unit of time. It is a good idea to have, at least, one set of changes in the laundry, one on the bed and one or more on the shelf. There is disagreement among facilities relating to how often, and under what circumstances, are bed linens actually changed. It is best to keep the responsibility for linen inventories, distribution, storage and washing in the hands of the laundry department. There are a variety of industry standards that can be utilized to test productivity. These tests of productivity will allow you to make the traditional comparison between laundry done in-house and laundry done on the contract basis. Whether you intend to contract laundry out through a private laundry or not, it is advisable to do a very detailed cost comparison between the two approaches to linen service. It is important to do this cost comparison because the question continually will come up—can the nursing home's laundry do a more cost effective job than an outside contractor—or can it not?

Maintenance Department

The maintenance department in most nursing homes usually consists of one person; a very versatile and experienced individual. Rarely will you find someone who is a qualified civil engineer. These are often individuals who have worked in hotels, hospitals, light industry or the military. They rarely have a degree, but are often one of the most reliable persons in the facility.

The maintenance person should be responsible for minor carpentry, electrical and plumbing work, and be able to figure out most minor building maintenance problems. He should have a good working knowledge and the ability to work with major hospital systems, such as water, electricity, and power.

Often it is advisable to call in outside contractors, who work at higher technical levels in plumbing, electrical, carpentry, etc., higher than those that are possessed by the maintenance man. It is important that both he and the administrator share an awareness of his limitations, and be able to agree on the advisability of getting outside help when really necessary.

Most nursing homes have numerous outside contract services that should be monitored and developed by the maintenance man with the administrator's assistance. For example, a service contract for dishwashing machines or other kitchen equipment; a service contract for the fire alarm system, for laundry machine maintenance; for elevators. All of these are very common. Pest control contracts, routine preventive maintenance and/or repair of medical equipment and call signal maintenance contracts are usually needed as well.

With the maintenance man, additional in-service training is as necessary as it is with other departments. The maintenance man should have a good sense of energy and energy conservation, and of how to do minor remodeling. The maintenance man should be very knowledgeable about safety and sanitation, and should be or become familiar with both state and federal regulations in this area. If the maintenance man has any ability at all, he will develop a preventive maintenance program for motors, pumps, electrical switches, lighting, etc., which will be a definite economic saving to the facility. Acute hospitals have very good in-service training for their maintenance staff. Often in an acute hospital the director of maintenance is an engineer or highly qualified person. It would be a good idea for the administrator of a skilled nursing facility to see if his maintenance man can take part in in-service training at a nearby acute hospital, even if cost is involved: it will be well worth the investment.

In larger facilities, the maintenance man may have an assistant who does a variety of tasks, which will include errands, operating garbage disposal units, loading trucks and vehicles, etc. Since physical plant and equipment have a tendency to break down outside of normal business hours, it would be important to have a maintenance man who is willing and able to come in at all hours of the night (with appropriate financial compensation). The maintenance man must also be able to deal with and communicate equitably with the many outside contractors mentioned above.

Another very important component of the maintenance program is to develop a list of priority calls. Since the maintenance man will no doubt be inundated with repair and maintenance requests in quantities that give him a backlog at all times, it would be very important to establish a list of circumstances that would be considered emergency or top priority, that must be done immediately. Some of these kinds of emergency maintenance relate to any situation where life would be endangered, such as a malfunctioning call system, an exposed electrical wire or an immediate fire hazard. The second level of priority usually relates to routine repairs in patient care areas and the third level of priority relates to routine repair in non-patient care or support areas. Items at the fourth level of priority are usually quite minor and in quite an abundance. Long-term projects, which will be ongoing, include preventive maintenance, record keeping and construction and remodeling planning.

The two most common problems that develop between the maintenance man and the other departments are the way he prioritizes their requests and the speed at which the requests are responded to. Quite clearly, the establishment of the priority schedule I just mentioned is an important factor in alleviating and reducing these potential interdepartmental conflicts. While the maintenance function operates, apparently, behind the scenes, if it is not carried out there can be a serious impairment not only in the overall function of the institution, but in the ambiance of the environment. We have already defined the importance of the environment in rendering care to patients, and impacting visitor attitude. If the heat is not working, if a light is malfunctioning, if furnishings are broken down, etc., then we can consider the environment itself to have failed to support the quality of life needs of the residents.

If the facility takes advantage of automation, certain programs within the maintenance department can be developed and kept on an ongoing basis with a limited amount of resources. For example, there are software packages for preventive maintenance groups. There is a quality assurance monitoring program appropriate for larger facilities. There are ways to schedule and maintain the variety of contracts we referred to, and a program to be used to cost out the energy utilization and required regulatory documentation. It is not really necessary to have a maintenance man who is knowledgeable in automation, if the administrator to whom the maintenance man reports utilizes these reports to govern maintenance performance.

The most useful tool in organizing the maintenance man's day is to devise a system that reduces his decisions as to which project to work on.

The top priority should be those projects that are listed as emergencies, and they would fall in the category of problems that endanger life or situations that could endanger life or create an emergency if not treated. Other work order requests could be described in terms of the timeliness needed to complete the job. One recommendation would be to divide the remaining work orders into those that must be done within 4 hours, those that must be done within 8 hours, those that are routine and can be delayed if necessary, and those that are long term, possibly part of a preventive maintenance program.

Preventive maintenance programs minimize long-term maintenance costs. The astute administrator will find some way to generate resources for this extremely cost-effective program.

MEDICAL RECORDS DEPARTMENT

While some of the larger facilities have the luxury of having a medical records librarian, either a registered record administrator or an Accredited Record Technician (ART), most nursing homes usually train a clerical person to become the medical records technician, whether they become certified or not. They then contract out the more sophisticated medical record services to an RRA or ART. These individuals work on a contract basis and supervise the activities of the in-house personnel.

Given the importance of the medical record function to the smooth operation of the nursing home, it is quite surprising how few resources we invest in making it run properly. Normally, outside consultants are restricted to very tight timelines, which consist of monitoring the work of the records tech, auditing medical records in a random sampling basis, and giving the key staff (primarily nursing) in-service training.

Larger corporations have the advantage of hiring highly skilled people to serve two or more facilities in this capacity and therefore, very often, the corporate chains are able to demonstrate greater levels of competency in the maintenance of medical records. As we know, a great deal of regulatory compliance is based on accuracy of medical records and related documents. Therefore, some investment of administrative activity in this area is crucial to addressing the needs of the regulatory process.

As stated before, the two most sought after credentials, as independent contractors, are the registered record administrator (RRA), usually obtained after receiving a 4-year degree; and the accredited record technician (ART), usually obtained through a 2-year or community college program. Both of these professions require a certain amount of on the job or clinical experience, and an examination by a national organization. Even though medical records in a skilled nursing facility are not as complex as the acute hospital, the basic functions that take place in an acute hospital must be duplicated. For example, the following records must be processed: admissions, discharge, transcription of orders, coding, abstracting, correspondence and storage.

The in-house record technician must be trained to perform an audit and prepare medical records for the more thorough examination that takes place during the periodic visit of the contract RRA or ART. It is very useful to have this records tech at the UR meetings. Since the success of the medical records system at the nursing home rests not only with the capability of the record tech and the contract consultant, but with the method of organizing, we should be aware that there are variety of methods of assembling records and numbering them.

Additionally, there are different types of filing systems and indexing systems, all of which have had a great deal of research done on them to support their value. The good record consultant will no doubt select the traditional methods of systematizing, numbering and indexing medical records for the average nursing home. Since we now have automated systems that work on microcomputers that automate admission, discharge and transfers, and many other of the medical records functions, we can obtain a higher level of accuracy and immediacy in the completion of medical records. At the same time, the audit process can be more efficient and more utilitarian for the administration.

In order for the medical records technician to succeed, the administration must give strong support to the technician's efforts to assure that all parties cooper ate in completing the medical records in a timely manner. If the medical record tech does not have this support, one can be assured that the records will not be completed on time, and that many problems will be unearthed during the next inspection. One only needs to review the numerous requirements that exist to realize the incredible importance of documentation and the maintenance of accurate and credible medical records.

THERAPEUTIC ACTIVITIES

We deal with the essentials of therapeutic activities in the discussion of the psychosocial model and the medical model. In the traditional medical model the activities program was a support to the rehabilitation function of the skilled nursing facility, and as such usually concentrated on the traditional programs of bingo, birthday and crafts (BBC). When we then extended the model to the psychosocial concept, we expanded the activities program to be a major component of the managed environment, and in this case BBC became strictly an adjunct to the health services intervention that supported the managed environment. While the substance of the activity program addressed involvement therapy, motivation therapy, reality orientation, somewhat new modalities were also introduced—such as yoga, meditation and massage, and a full array of creative and growth-oriented programming.

It is quite clear that the Activity Director of today must not only be better trained, but must view his position as a much more significant contributor to the patient well-being than ever before. In those states that have mandated positions officially called activity director or therapeutic activity director, there is usually a concurrent requirement for licensing or certification. While the position rarely requires a bachelor degree or a master's degree specialty in therapeutic activities, some form of training program, at least on the community college level, is warranted. Unfortunately, even with the more enlightened approach taken by many states in defining the responsibility of the activities person in a skilled nursing home, very little time is allocated to this immensely important resource. I've often used the expression "activities department," when in fact, the department is usually one individual who, in a 100 bed facility, will not normally work full time. If this is the case, i.e., that you have approximately 40 hours of activity worker per 100 beds, then we must take a very close look at how this person uses his time while in the facility. The most obvious problem that develops is that this person spends a great deal of time with one on one activities, which automatically means that the activity director must neglect others, who will not receive activities. In other words where there are very limited resources in the activities department, ways must be developed to maximize the benefits from every hour that the individual works in the hospital. Recalling the psychosocial model, more of the activity workers time should be allocated to mobilizing community and family references. Secondly, group activities should be emphasized over individual ones. I believe that with the limited amount of resources, represented by the activity worker, more time should be allocated to mobilizing community and family resources, and to assist in maximizing the activity worker's very limited time by emphasizing group activities. Therefore people will not be arbitrarily triaged out of any program because of the bias of the institution, the staff or the activity worker. One of the regulatory requirements that is quite consistent throughout the states is that of documentation of activity therapy assessments, activity plans, as well as recording attendance at these various activities.

The burden that falls on the activity worker is usually quite heavy, because there is very little time and very much that must be done for the overall well-being of the resident population. In recent years there are new methods of developing greater positive family involvement in the activities of the patient and of the facility as a whole, through family nights, family councils, and structured staff and family programs.

The development of involvement programming, such as resident council (mandated in most states), menu committees, hostess committees, and other group functions, again multiplies the impact of every hour of activity worker service. The activity worker must be an active member of the patient care planning committee, and must be able to contribute to the deliberations of care programming at all levels of the nursing home operations.

Sometimes this responsibility is handled by a social worker, a chaplain, an occupational therapist or a specialist in therapeutic activities. When the nursing home has the opportunity to have people with these higher levels of skills, there is also the opportunity of raising the overall quality of life at the facility. The administrator must support this function of therapeutic activities wholeheartedly, even to the extent of actively participating in family nights, community home functions and the development of volunteer programs.

It is hoped that the tremendous value of the therapeutic activity worker is realized at some time in the future and the miserly approach to doling out small amounts of this time dispensed with. Next to the increased ratios of more assistants to the residents, it is imperative that more therapeutic activity workers be added to the nursing home community.

Business Office

The Business Office of the Nursing Home performs the following primary services:

1. patient trust fund account management
2. accounts payable
3. accounts receivable
4. payroll
5. personnel management
6. budgeting
7. petty cash control
8. financial statements
9. fiscal audit
10. insurance portfolio management

The Business Office is usually led by someone called the Office Manager who normally is a person who has trained as a billing clerk and has evolved through the system and picked up a great deal of knowledge about bookkeeping. Many Office Managers have several years of college and occasionally there will be some with college degrees in some form of fiscal management. The diversity of services required by the nursing home business office is unusual. Even in the acute hospital, the business office and accounting office are separated. Because all of the functions mentioned above take place in one small environment, it should be the focus of great administrative interest on a day-to-day business. While the Office or Business Manager is the top person in this department who must report to the Administrator, the staffing pattern usually consists of one or more billing clerks and a clerical person. If I had to place in the top priority one of their assignments, the collection of receivables would be head and shoulders above all other duties.

The collection of the bills owed to the hospital is surprisingly complex and the procedure for assuring that revenue is brought into the facility in a timely manner has a variety of steps. Many people consider the Medicaid billing system in the nursing home field to be one of the most difficult billing systems of any field. The slightest error in timing, the slightest misstatement of diagnoses or a delayed approval at one point or another could mean a substantial delay in repayment or total denial of the bill. I will not be going into the full program for Medicaid, Medicare and third party billing. But, it should be noted that many administrators lose their jobs by virtue of their inability to collect their bills in a timely manner. The loss or delay of revenue has a devastating effect on a tightly-managed nursing home. I have been a consultant to many facilities where the primary problem was the inability to collect their bills resulting in an unacceptable level of accounts receivable. Many business office managers have gotten their positions by virtue of their ability to develop a very tight billing program that ensures speedy return of revenues. Facilities that have unacceptably high levels of accounts receivable will invariably have other fiscal problems. I have noted a pattern between a high level of accounts receivable and a high level of accounts payable for obvious reasons, if they don't get the money in they are not going to be paying their bills. Once a nursing home has a problem of not paying their bills, a variety of other issues develop. For example, purveyors not paid in a timely manner may withhold delivery. Sometimes employees paychecks are not ready on payday which is very damaging to employee morale, and so on.

Another vitally important aspect of the business office function is the maintenance of the patient trust fund accounts. These monies must be kept in a demand trust available to the resident upon request. There must not only be documentation of all expenditures out of this trust; but, a periodic (usually quarterly) reporting of the balance of these reports must be rendered to the patient in a timely manner. The management of the patient trust money is so important that it should be of primary concern to the administrator who must develop a monitoring program that assures total compliance with all laws and regulations. This program must incorporate an outside third party auditor at appropriate times. A business office function is the appropriate disbursement of funds of the deceased residents. This must be done with a great deal of finesse. It is not uncommon for relatives who did not have a legal responsibility for the resident to attempt to receive the deceased resident's valuables. There are very specific rules and regulations governing the disbursement of deceased persons' funds and they should be followed explicitly.

One of the advantages of multi-facility ownership is the centralizing of the billing office functions, which decreases the unit expense of this administrative department as the nursing home chain gets larger. The chains of nursing homes with three or more facilities often have centralized business offices with all of the functions mentioned above fully computerized. This offers the opportunity to intensely monitor all of these functions and will give the administrator a variety of information upon which to make management decisions.

Business offices, even in small nursing homes, are automated to some degree. The kind of things a computer will usually do is to: (1) post charges to patient accounts and monitor these accounts (2) generate bills and automatically issue collection statements to patients, and (3) maintain the budget and produce monthly profit and loss statements that may be monitored.

These are but a few of the many functions in a business office that can be monitored.

Some of the most typical business office problems are:

1. late charges from ancillary services
2. unacceptably high levels of bad debt write-off
3. high accounts receivable

4. slow cash flow
5. inaccurate discharge information
6. inaccurate data on billing forms

A very important analytic tool that must be produced either manually or by computer is the aged receivable. The aged receivable is a breakdown of the bills, usually in thirty, sixty and ninety days and older that lets you know of the success of your collection procedure. Another formula often used is measuring the accounts receivable by the number of days outstanding. Days outstanding is usually defined as the amount of outstanding revenue divided by the revenue average per day. The aged receivable is a more useful process to help you deal with potentially serious collection problems and reconcile the receivables with collection of bad debt in a timely manner. Receivables may be evaluated by any of the following dimensions:

1. by account
2. by volume of accounts
3. by the value of dollars
4. by source (i.e., Medicare, Medicaid, etc.)
5. by the aging I've just described

A variety of other functions in the business office lend themselves to specialized analyses. Analyses such as time flow for the billing process and the systems connected with it. Secondly, a credit and collection analysis which studies among other things, bad debt and the effectiveness of collection procedures. Another analytical tool would be one that gives an indepth review of accounts payable which includes control and verification of bills received. In other words, the administrator has many devices to monitor the function of the business office. All of them must be used for successful financial management.

RETURN ON INVESTMENT

A well-run proprietary hospital will develop standards for return on investment which takes gross revenues less projected operating costs to produce a projected net income.

Gross income is usually derived from historical data, or, for new facilities, or budget projections. These take into account: (1) the number of patients and their funding mix (public assistance vs. private pay), and (2) their length of stay and acuity levels. The patient days in each category then are multiplied by the projected reimbursement for that category to produce the gross projected revenues.

This type of well-run hospital also has internal operating standards that tightly control expenses in each particular area. For example, in laundry they will have a rigid control of pounds per patient day and a tightly controlled cost per pound of laundry. They will have labor costs broken out by nursing hours (cost per patient day) and all other labor costs per patient day. They will also have projected food costs per patient day. The total of these standardized, tightly managed cost factors equals the operating expense for that facility for any projected period of time. We then take the projected gross revenues less these projected operating expenses and are able to end up with a projected net income. The administrator of the facility is responsible for meeting these standards of projected net income. Usually, if net income is not met, the cause is in the census of the hospital or the patient mix which shows less private pay than projected in the original gross income projections. Profit margins are determined by the expenses that are deducted from the original net income such as taxes, capital payback, etc.

Because business office personnel communicate on a daily basis with residents and their families, it is important that their communications skills be considered an important factor when hiring. It is also wise to augment this basic communication skill by specialized training and continuous reinforcement of the need for the business office to act as a positive representative of the nursing home. Business office workers often consider the resident interaction as one of the more important parts of their daily work; so this relationship, even though it is business-oriented can become a very supportive process for both resident and office worker.

PARAMEDICAL SERVICES

While chains or large nursing homes may have salaried paramedical personnel, most skilled nursing facilities receive these services by contract. For example, the following services are normally contracted out with different combinations of monthly retainers and fee-for-service billings:

1. occupational therapy
2. physical therapy
3. speech therapy
4. radiology
5. laboratory
6. pharmacy consultation
7. dietetic consultation
8. medical records consultation
9. dental consultation
10. podiatry consultation
11. vision services consultation

All of these support services should have a training responsibility to the staff of the facility. And, because of that must receive funding usually on an hourly basis for these special training programs. The billing for the services rendered to each individual resident is normally handled by the professional; but, may under some circumstances be handled through the nursing home's billing office. The administrator must be very careful to monitor the billing systems of each of these professionals to assure that the residents are not disadvantaged by their billing programs. There are very stringent Medicare and Medicaid guidelines that govern the vast majority of paramedical service billings and these should be strictly adhered to and monitored very closely. The interrelationship between private payment for these paramedical services and payment received from third party payors must be looked at very closely to assure the residents that they will not be charged privately for a service that could or should be paid for by a third party payor. Even in the best of circumstances some element of confusion may result in these kinds of billing systems.

Whether these services are rendered by a proprietary organization or a nearby hospital, the contract must be reviewed and renewed each year.

PHYSICIAN SERVICES

The role of the Medical Director in the skilled nursing facility has been evolving for some time. During the early stages of the development of the field, the Medical Director was a titular position usually filled by a physician who had a certain number of patients in the facility. The primary functions of the Medical Director are to act as a liaison officer between the administrator and the attending physicians, and, to be in charge of reviewing both administrative and patient care policies and procedures. The Medical Director is the main consultant to the Director of Nurses as relates to patient care services and must also review the health of the employees ensuring that they have met the health criteria established by state and/or federal regulations for employment and for continued employment.

The Medical Director is also an excellent linkage between the facility and the medical community as well as an invaluable source of inservice education for different departments within the nursing home. Should there be a problem with the functioning of a primary physician, it is advisable to utilize the services of the Medical Director to intervene. State and federal regulations that govern the operation of the nursing home usually do not relate to the clinical practice of medicine which is often covered by a separate medical practices act. While the administration is responsible for those components of medical practice relating to services required under regulations, they are not responsible for the clinical aspects of the practice of medicine. It is very important in terms of understanding the relation of survey and compliance procedures, to recognize the difference between the clinical practice of medicine and the administrative support structure that enables the physician to practice in the facility. Whether a particular component of the doctor's function is the administrator's responsibility or that of the physician is often the subject of some debate and even litigation. For example, should a physician not complete his legally-required medical record documentation, it is the nursing home's responsibility to remind him. And, this responsibility is not abated until a procedure to remind the physician in an appropriate fashion is completed. After the hospital's responsibility in initiating this reminder is completed, it will then become the physician's liability should the record not be completed and therefore be reviewed under the medical practices act as a clinical issue and not an administrative issue. This fine line must be monitored very carefully and the

Medical Director is often an excellent judge as to when the line has been crossed and the issue is no longer the responsibility of the hospital administration. In their capacities as physicians, Medical Directors can also deal with problems that develop with the clinical practice of medicine within the guidelines established by the medical profession.

Patients may only be admitted to a skilled nursing facility by the direct order of a physician and be under the care of a physician selected by the patient or the patient's representative. The attending physician will be responsible for completing a physical examination either immediately before or after admission. The doctor is also responsible for the patient diagnosis(ses), written orders for diet and care, diagnostic tests, treatments and medications. The attending physician will render important advice in terms of the overall care plan and of the appropriate level of care needed for the patient and will provide for an alternative physician during times of unavailability.

The hospital is responsible for making arrangements for emergency medical care if either the attending physician or designee is not available.

Non-physician practitioners of a variety of kinds may practice those services for which they are legally authorized and licensed to perform. For example, a physician's assistant or nurse practitioner working under the responsibility and supervision of a physician is an acceptable practice in most states. Other forms of healers and health practitioners who may not have legal sanction for their practice normally do not render services in nursing homes. The physician must offer continuing supervision of the patient and evaluate that individual at least every thirty days unless there is a documented program that allows longer periods between these evaluations.

The Medical Director when discharging responsibility for the development of bylaws, the rules and regulations that govern patient care policies and procedures, also delineates the responsibilities of the attending physician. The Medical Director evaluates the clinical practice of medicine, as well as the functioning of paramedical support services. While most Medical Directors are retained by the facilities as independent contractors, those facilities that have organized medical staff usually have a Medical Director designated by that group with the approval of the governing body or ownership of the facility. Sometimes the Medical Director is acquired through arrangement with a local group of physicians, a medical society, or nearby hospital medical staff through a similar contractual relationship. There are many questions concerning malpractice and related liability concerns, so the definition of the relationship, i.e., independent contractor vs. employee, is often of considerable importance. Whether the Medical Director also has patients within the facility, and, the relationship of their own malpractice insurance premiums to the new responsibility are often important points in the negotiations with a potential Medical Director.

Departmental Functions

PUTTING IT ALL TOGETHER

In this chapter we have described departmental functions, and have attempted to cover all of the most commonly accepted components of a skilled nursing facility. This, however, does not really tell the story. Because the phenomena that occurs is that the whole is much greater than the sum of its parts. The synergistic workings of these departments creates, or should create, a total institutional culture. Toward these ends we must acknowledge that the components of the psycho-social model, the family and community involvement, are a necessary component to what the total institutional culture is.

For many years, the idea of a resident council has been proposed as one component of the managed environment. It is my opinion that the resident council as currently structured is only a part of the total institutional culture of a managed environment.

The more successful concept, in my opinion, has been the regenerative community which does not have the structured hierarchical leadership, but which relies on a communal, egalitarian structure for the generation of a quality environment. Its integration of the staff worker assures his or her role as resident advocate. Its lack of reliances on time-limited leadership allows much greater stability and longevity. This concept should be developed to a much greater extent.

In either case, whether it's the traditional resident council or the regenerative community (sometimes these can work in a complementary fashion), the hidden factor is that there must be professional staff leadership to create these entities and maintain them as ongoing benefits for the resident community.

The resident council is an organizational structure within the resident population that elects a president, other officers and special committees that are run by the residents themselves. If a facility has very few people at the degree of alertness needed to exercise leadership, then the resident council ceases to be a functional unit that assures residents' needs are being expressed. On the other hand, if the organization has many very alert people, the extreme result of a very "successful" resident council could be the creation of an adversarial group that is unreasonable in its relationship with staff and management. This is seldom an improvement.

I am of the opinion that the idea of the regenerative community should start at the very earliest level of socializing networks that the elderly have access to, such as senior centers or senior housing, and that the implementation of such organizations only at the nursing home stage is incomplete and much more difficult to accomplish. While I support the merits of resident structures, I think that much work has to be done to design such structures to assure that they benefit the entire institutional community and are able to have an ongoing positive impact on the quality of life of the individual resident.

MULTI-LEVEL FACILITIES

Multi-level facilities are primarily found in the nonprofit sector of the long term care system. The two most common combinations of service levels are skilled nursing and residential care. The second most frequent combination is independent living and residential care. Some facilities have a broader spectrum of institutional services offering residential care; intermediate and skilled care; or intermediate, residential and skilled care. Some organizations have the entire continuum located on one campus, where a continuity of service is offered between independent living, residential, intermediate care and skilled nursing. In some cases, acute units are also part of these larger multi-level institutions. If there is any variety in the proprietary facility, it is in combinations of intermediate care and skilled nursing, with skilled nursing predominating.

Multi-level organizations, and even more particularly those that have continuing or life care contracts are obligated to supply most services in the continuum. Many management problems ensue from the complex service delivery matrix that exists in such closed systems. For example, depending on the state, the delivery of certain health services into a non health system may be against state regulations. A case could be made for considering personal care units that receive an exceptionally high degree of nursing servies as de facto nursing units. This would lead one to conclude that the resident in that particular unit is a bonafide nursing candidate and should not be there in the first place. The management of this form of long term care facility is therefore complicated by these interactions. Additional to the care-oriented problems described, one normally finds a variety of ownership and turf problems that one does not usually encounter in one level service systems.

For example, when an elderly person lives for some length of time in one particular unit of the facility, and then must be transferred to another unit because of the need for a higher level of service, there is often an unwillingness on his and the part of his family to encourage and support that move. Concurrent with this unwillingness to move is the demand that other services be brought to the resident.

Since most of the residents of these multi-level facilities are upper middle income people, the ability to demand service and attention (from a political viewpoint) is much higher than the comparable ability of a lower economic group. And therefore, one could assume that the management of multi-level facilities will be difficult from these many viewpoints. When we realize that these organizations are primarily (although not exclusively) nonprofit, we must also take into account the existence of a board of directors and recognize that the administrators relationship to the board of directors is in itself part of the art form of management. When effecting the movement of either services or individuals within a multi-level system, the manager needs to demonstrate a high degree of tact and diplomacy in dealing not only with the state regulatory bodies, but, also with the internal needs and demands of the resident population and, most probably, with the oversight demands of a board of directors.

MAKING THE CONTINUUM WORK

We have described the integral components of a conceptual continuum of care based on meeting the needs of a frail elderly person. The continuum is designed with one goal in mind: to help the individual maintain maximum social and physical independence, and consequently, as high a quality of life as their circumstances allow. There are certain processes that are necessary to make this continuum operative.

ASSESSMENT

Through a procedure called assessment, the needs of the person are determined. The assessment process may be abbreviated or quite in-depth. Once the assessment is concluded, a care plan is developed indicating the services needed in terms of quantity, quality, time and economic limitations.

CASE MANAGEMENT

Case management is a process that implements the care plan, monitors its success, evaluates the outcomes, and then modifies the plan as needed. Elderly sometimes do not like the concept of case management because they do not like to be "managed." Nevertheless, the process described under the rubric of case management is necessary to prevent the elderly from "falling in between the cracks" of the particular system that exists. Long term care is not an integrated and coordinated system at this time, and the glue that may be the integrating factor is case management. The case manager, who usually follows direction from a multidisciplinary team may come from a variety of disciplines . . . nursing, medicine or social services being the most common. There are many definitions of the term which has recently become a fixture in human service lexicon.

Channeling

Channeling is the function that directs the elderly person on a certain course of action. It will map out the linked series of services that the elderly person should receive. Since these discrete services are normally independent of each other, the process of channeling often is impaired because of the particular vested interest approach of each of these components of the service network. The implied integration of services that would expedite the channeling process has yet to be realized.

Access

Another function of case management which occurs after the channeling process is that of accessing the individual into the particular service. The problem of access has many barriers, including lack of resources, lack of financial support, or case specific limitations. The essence of access is getting the older person into a service. The skill of the case manager in overcoming these access barriers is the main determinant of the quality of this particular service.

Another aspect of the case management approach is economic, in that most case managers assume the role of the economic manager of the care plan. It is the case manager's responsibility to assure that the varied economic problems encountered by the elderly recipient are resolved. In certain model projects, where the care plan must be funded by a capitated system, the case manager assumes a crucial role in making economic decisions that may conflict with the imperatives of the care that was needed.

The role of case manager has become pivotal in the success of the continuum of care, and it will occupy a crucial position in the development of the long term care system. Training of this individual thus far has been done on a project by project basis. There are no uniform standards academically, educationally or empirically. It will be one of the challenges of the future to design case management as a separate distinct profession of its own with standards and accreditation where appropriate.

Problems in the Continuum of Care

The continuum of care as described above is an ideal and does not exist in reality. The most common result of the lack of a truly integrated service system is the arbitrary shuffling of the elderly person between home, hospital, and nursing home. Since the concepts of assessment, case management and continuum of care are not generally accepted, those responsible for determining the care received by the elderly, or assisting the elderly in making their own care decisions, simply refer the elderly to a nursing home. This is the most common and predominant component of long term care. In terms of the acute hospital's continuity of care, or progressive patient care, the nursing home is the most visible and readily available component of the continuum, and therefore the end of the line for many elderly leaving the acute hospital system. Since the people who are making the discharge decisions are usually hospital-oriented, and since those assisting the elderly in dealing with their needs at home are also medically-oriented, there is little room for the implementation or development of the continuum beyond this triangle which routes the elderly again and again from home to hospital to nursing home.

This problem is magnified by planners in government whose only knowledge of long term care is the nursing home. Many financial constructs of broad scale government programs will, because of this shortsightedness, relate to this same triangle. Integrated continuums exist in certain model projects, but because of this lack of oversight planning will not significantly impact the system.

Another problem in the development of the integrated continuum is that it must be preceded by sound demographic forecasting. Once the thorough demographic study is completed and a needs analysis is produced, the types and magnitudes of specific services can be designed into the system. Unfortunately merely designing them into the system doesn't create them, and we find—because each service in a community could be sponsored by a different interest group—that the development of special resources to support an integrated continuum may be difficult, if not impossible. For example, if it is noted that a major problem in the continuum is a lack of senior housing, the timeline between this realization and the actual opening of the doors of a senior housing project may be many years. Difficulties encountered in the interim in developing needed resources are magnified precisely because of this gap. We find that because the needs analysis of any given population changes as the population changes, the decisions made originally to provide resources to meet the needs of the continuum must also change.

The fastest utilization of resources are primarily those that are programmatic and do not require brick and mortar. Conversely, the slowest implementation of resources are those that require capital investment.

Another complexity is that many resources are created by community effort, a long arduous process of involving community groups and motivating them to support the initiation of a particular project, such as a day care center, a senior center, home meal program and so on.

A final barrier to the successful development of the continuum of care is the lack of economic resources. A large percentage of the money in the long term care system goes to support the nursing home component and consequently little is allocated to the variety of other services, despite the fact that these others, if functioning properly (i.e., *funded* properly) could reduce overall need for institutional care. Senior centers in outreach organizations are all marginally funded and have severe limitations on the number of services they are able to render to the elderly and those few individual services that are adequately funded very often are incorporated into the ever-expanding proprietary health care delivery system.

MODELS OF DELIVERY

There are a variety of methods one can use to analyze how we deliver services. Dialogues, schematics, linear definitions, and information trees are some techniques often used.

A most effective technique in describing delivery of long term care services is to develop a model of delivery that utilizes in its schematic the various components of the delivery system and links these various components in the delivery system by function, direction, and the definition of the end product. The model should indicate what the "drive" is, so that the moving force of the delivery system is indicated quite clearly. Thus, we have all the factors that are utilized in the delivery of service of long term care.

The Medical Model

Referencing our discussion of the historical evolution of the long term care system, we note that the modern nursing home began its relationship with the acute hospitals sometime during the early 1950s. At this stage of evolution, the nursing home was viewed as the place where discharges from the acute hospitals went to live out the rest of their days. And as time went on, the regulations that evolved for the skilled nursing facility were quite clearly derivative of the acute hospital regulations. Not only were similar definitions used for the various levels of personnel, but also for the variety of standards, physical plant designs and other regulatory characteristics.

It is therefore quite logical to assume that the design of the nursing home would follow what we will call the medical model of delivery.

As would be anticipated, the medical model of delivery is doctor centered, as is the acute hospital. Therefore the "drive" of the entire delivery system is the physician. The physician functions through the medical diagnosis, which is converted into the doctor's orders, and the doctor's orders drive the entire system from then on. The doctor's orders request very specialized services such as laboratory, x-ray. They also direct the nursing staff and paramedical staff on a course of action to deal with the pathology that has been diagnosed. This design for the medical model was formulated in the late 1930s when hospitals emerged as the physicians' workshop, and the centralization of medical practice became a reality in the health scene. Prior to this formalization of the acute medical model most medicine was practiced in the patient's home. If one were to analyze the hospitals in olden times, one would find that they were primarily for the poor, and that the wealthier people were cared for entirely at home until the emergence of this acute model during the '30s.

The medical model we use now, however, is not the acute medical model, but a simplified version that represents the model upon which skilled nursing services were derived. Unlike the acute medical model, the doctor's orders are then converted into three primary modalities. The first is medication, the second is treatment, and the third rehabilitation. Medication, in the medical model for the skilled nursing facility is primary treatment modality. While the quantity of medications rendered to the elderly residents is very high, the variety of these medications is much more limited than those prescribed for a patient in an acute hospital. One of the interesting characteristics of the population we are caring for is the unfortunately large number of medications they may take at home. It is not unusual to see a patient admitted into a skilled nursing facility consuming 8-14 different medications. (Granted, some of these may be over the counter.) What we find in the nursing home is that this situation is replicated in that most nursing home patients are on many routine medications.

The primary medications given are for restraint purposes. Study after study of the nursing home population has revealed an excessive use of medications in order to make the patient more malleable and easier for the staff to care for. The large amount of control medications used has been under close scrutiny for many years, and it is the goal of many farsighted people to reduce the importance of this form of medication and to shift the burden of behavioral modification to more positive and successful approaches.

The second modality, treatments, consists of a whole spectrum of services done to the patient by a great number of nursing and paramedical support staff. This consists of the full gamut of bedside nursing treatments, therapeutic diets, podiatric services, dental services, etc. It is a most familiar modality, because here again it parallels quite closely that which happens in an acute hospital.

The third direct modality is rehabilitation. It consists of those services that are offered by physical therapists, occupational therapists, speech therapists, and other health professionals. The goal of the rehabilitation portion is to improve the individual's function to a point where further rehabilitative services are no longer needed. Specifically, this is accomplished by addressing rehabilitative needs that are directly related to the cause of admission to the skilled nursing services or related to those functions that will allow the patient to be discharged back into the community. These standards are derivative of Medicare standards, which tightly govern the use of rehabilitative services.

As an adjunct to rehabilitative services, we have what we euphemistically call "activities." These are presented by trained activity workers, and, at least, consist of the famous "BBC": birthday, bingo and crafts, for which nursing homes are so well noted. These activities are usually an afterthought, and about 1% of the total operating budget is allocated towards activities.

These three major modalities fit into a patient care plan that is monitored and updated as needed. The updating of this patient care plan is the responsibility, from a professional standpoint, of the director of nurses, and is usually carried out by the charge nurse on the particular unit the patient is in. The review of the patient care plan is most intense on the regulatory level, but because of the time needed to maintain these documents, most facilities fall short in executing them properly.

Describing the model thus far, we have a doctor centered structure that uses the doctor's orders as the primary moving device and which concentrates on three primary modalities of service: medications, treatments, and physical rehabilitation; activities being a support for rehabilitation. What then would be the goal of this model? Of necessity we must reflect on the goal of the acute hospital, which is the patient's physical well-being. Since the average length of stay in the acute hospital is between six and eight days, a great deal of high technology must be brought to bear on the pathology that caused the admission. Therefore the goal of this medical model must be physical well-being. By the same token, this is the goal in the skilled nursing home. However, while physical well-being is a plus, and a commendable goal for a nursing home, we must recognize that in the population we are discussing, chronic illnesses preclude, in many cases, healing or reversals of certain conditions. In point of fact, physical well-being may be interpreted as preventing rapid regression.

The issue of whether this goal of physical well-being is reality based gave many thinkers in the late part of the 1960s concern and encouraged the evolution of a different model of delivery of services in the skilled nursing facility.

During these years, the climate in the long term care field was directed towards public concern over the quality of care in nursing homes. Throughout the country headlines promulgated horror stories that spurred investigations and rethinking of the regulatory process that governed the nursing home. For the first time, the sense that community attitude was a factor in the quality assurance of these facilities was established. While the emphasis of the public concern appeared to be directed at poor regulations and poor enforcement of the existing relations, another less visible scenario emerged.

This interesting new viewpoint dealt with those facilities that were giving good or excellent care. It was noted that in many of these facilities the public clamor was no less than for those facilities that gave bad care. This led to the conclusion that even under the most optimal circumstances the end product or goal of the medical model could meet all standards and regulations of the regulatory bodies and yet not be acceptable to the community, patients, and families.

What then could be concluded? Primarily that the goal of physical well-being could not be successful even under the most optimal of circumstances; that the medical model designed after the acute hospital was inappropriate for the long term care patient, and could be applied successfully only to a relatively small percent of those who were admitted to the skilled nursing facility. Part of this analysis took into account that each patient received less than 3 hours of direct care on an average of any 24-hour day. The rest of this 24-hour day the patient was under observation. This figure of direct service was a combination of all of the treatments, rehabilitative services and medications that were rendered the patient in a 24-hour period.

In order to construct a model that more accurately addresses the overall needs of the patient, we had to analyze what was lacking in the medical model, as well as address more generic problems faced by the frail or disabled elderly person. At first glance, the medical model, using the physician centered approach, probably lost the valuable input of a variety of other disciplines that could have contributed greatly to a broader analysis of the needs of the patient. If we accepted this viewpoint, we also had to recognize that both the medical diagnosis and the doctor's orders, which were integral in moving the model, would no longer be acceptable. We had to address the reality that the utilization of medications, which was a primary method of care, was greatly flawed in that its emphasis on control medicines could be viewed as a negative. We looked at these forms of chemical restraints as self-serving the staff of the facility and having questionable value in improving the life of the patient.

The second modality of delivery consisting mostly of basic patient care, and contingent treatments, emphasized sickness and disability. It perpetuated the medical model's effort to make the patient dependent upon service, and we felt this dependency was bad.

The third modality of service addressed rehabilitation only as it related to the Medicare standards of reimbursement, and therefore did not address a variety of rehabilitative modes that could enhance the patients' well-being. The augmentation of the rehabilitative services with limited traditional recreational activities was viewed as a minimalist approach to deal with an area of great concern.

MODELING TO MEET THE NEEDS:
THE PSYCHOSOCIAL MODEL

What we needed then was not just a critique of the acute medical model, but an analysis of the needs of the recipient of services in such a manner that the model would be designed to address these needs.

We found that the most significant characteristic of aging was that of multiple losses. The loss of being a wage earner, the loss of leadership in the family group, the loss of contact and the concurrent stimulation that one gets from being with and in touch with the community and family, the loss of dignity and self-esteem, the loss of independence, and the loss of the ability to learn and grow. We felt that if the model could be developed to somehow help the patient regain these losses, we would be on the right track in developing the goal of the truly successful model of delivery.

To start developing our model, we agreed that the physician who is trained to diagnosis and treat pathology must be part of the "drive" of the new model. Operationally, the physician, although the drive of the model, spent less than 20 minutes per month per patient (some say as little as 5 minutes per month per patient in many situations). This meant that the primary responsibility for delivery of service in the nursing home under the medical model was in reality the director of nurses. Many people feel that the medical model should actually be called the nursing model of care. In reality, this is just a malfunction of the medical model that relates to the very limited amount of MD time available for the patient. But what it did confirm was the need to have the RN involved as part of the drive. Further analysis led us to require an MSW, chaplain or gerontologist who had expert knowledge in the psychosocial and environmental and/or spiritual needs of the patient, and then an activity worker or other person who had knowledge of diversional or recreational needs. In essence we created a multi-faceted team, whose product would be the social diagnosis. This social diagnosis would be developed into a social program of which a sub-component would relate to the person's physical well-being.

To further address the needs of the elderly patient, we would implement the social program in a manner structurally similar to the medical model by developing three main modalities of care which converge to reach our ultimate goal.

FAMILY MODALITY

Elevating family involvement into the nursing home care as a major modality was our first step. In order to view the patient in the proper perspective, we viewed him or her as part of the family unit. We recognized that the exclusion of this family unit was a factor in the regressive cycle most elderly face. The support, the status, the respect that came from the family unit by and large was lost to the institutionalized individual and was a contributing factor to their isolation, loneliness, and loss of status. Considering family as a primary modality meant that this unit had to be addressed in a certain way. We found it a myth that American elderly are rejected by their family. Proper support techniques could bring the family and the institutionalized person closer together, and therefore the resources used in this effort were well worth it to replace the losses that the family's removal had created.

Special training programs have been developed to assist family members—sons, daughters, grandchildren—to have successful, positive visits by helping them overcome their own barriers when entering a nursing home. By giving them guidelines and encouragement they are often able to pull the older person back into the family unit.

COMMUNITY MODALITY

The second modality recognizes that the mentality that created the institutional model of delivery of service is an historical derivative of the mentality that excluded the elderly and disabled from society back in the days of the English poor laws. It recognizes that "out of sight out of mind" is a fact of life in society, and that the creation of the nursing home system is in some ways a response to that historical trend. We therefore create a treatment modality which assists in the process of "mainstreaming" and brings the person closer to the community from which he's been rejected.

This "bringing closer" process goes both ways. It means allocation of resources to develop volunteer programs with a patient population at large. It means organizing, on an individual basis, community linkages between a resident and some community resource that is recognized by them. It means reaffiliation in some cases with church, fraternal lodges, organizations, or neighbors. It means bringing those resources into the facility, and it means transporting the patient out into the community on a planned basis to link up in some manner with that community resource.

This community modality requires someone skilled in developing volunteer programs, organizing trips, developing community organized support groups, linking those support groups with both individuals and the patient population at large. This represents a fundamentally new skill in the skilled nursing facility.

GOAL OF THE NEW MODEL

We've now created a model of delivery that is multidisciplinary, team centered, uses a social program as its governing device and has three primary modalities. What do these lead to? In order to be consistent with our analysis of the medical model, we now have to develop a goal that could be the anticipated product to these three delivery modalities. One of the difficulties in developing such a goal is to come up with one that has some ability to be quantified. In essence, we did not want a goal that was nothing more than a euphemism or platitude. Nevertheless we chose to call our goal the *quality of life*, recognizing that the debate to determine the definition of quality of life will never end, and that we must, for the sake of our definition, select a half dozen criteria that made sense and that could, to some degree, be measured.

We reduce the risk in defining quality of care by using components of the definition that have some ability to be measured by current measurement tools in the field of human service.

Initially we must state that the primary component of the quality of life is physical well-being, because at no time does the psychosocial model deny the existence of the need for health or medically oriented services. Quite to the contrary; it acknowledges that physical well-being is part of quality of life, but it puts it in an entirely different perspective. Since we are choosing to consider physical well-being from a wellness concept versus a pathology concept, the physical well-being takes on a different perspective in that we are not primarily trying to heal pathology as much as we are trying to maximize physical potential. The dialogue on these interrelated viewpoints may go on indefinitely. In terms of our ability to manage the environment and achieve certain goals, however, it is the effort to deal with wellness and maximize potential that significantly reallocates our resources and redirects our thinking.

Consistent with the wellness concept, is the prevention of regression of physical capabilities while maximizing these physical potentials remaining to the older, disabled person. Therefore, while we use the same word, physical well-being, our emphasis on achieving this component of the goal is different than in the medical model.

Studies indicate that the most significant aspect of our psychosocial being is self-esteem. To the extent that any one characteristic is of primary importance in supporting longevity, self-esteem is viewed as that characteristic. Therefore, a major part of our quality of life is the existence of self-esteem and its maintenance and enhancement. Another characteristic that is in reality the same as self-esteem is dignity. While self-esteem may be an internally derived value, dignity is that same characteristic as bestowed upon that individual by another person. The managed environment, community and family, can therefore band together to both enhance the self-esteem and bestow dignity upon the individual.

Another characteristic of our definition of quality of life is the condition of independence. Note that we are not attempting to prevent dependence, which is often considered a meritorious goal, but we are consciously creating a situation that fosters independence. Institutional dependency is a phenomenon that we all observe, and unfortunately, it takes place very quickly, often within the first three months. Therefore, those factors that must come into play to create a situation of independence must be brought to bear on admission and carried forward in a methodological manner. Institutional dependence is quite insidious, and is often a significant barrier to rehabilitation and discharge. Many times the fear and uncertainties of independent living are reduced by institutional living to the point where the anticipation of again facing those fears is more than the resident wishes to do. And when services are, at some later date, removed in an effort to prevent further dependency, the resident will not be responsive.

The institutional dependency is a very strong force, unfortunately, if the independence concept is not implemented early on, it may never be successful. The elderly are quite resilient, and there is a sense of accommodation even under the worst of circumstances.

Another characteristic of our definition of quality of life is growth. This is probably one of the most difficult concepts to accept in its true definition. It is another example of a word that has a meaning that can be interpreted in terms of program, managed environment, and even measured outcome. One facet of growth is the encouragement of the development of goals. Now we may say what kind of goal can an 85-year-old institutionalized person have? Certainly the life goals as applied to younger and middle-aged people which relates to family and job and career may not be applicable in this case. There are, however, many kinds of goals that the institutionalized person could develop as part of a managed environment, and these goals are every bit as important to their quality of life as family and career are to younger people.

For example, let us take a most restrictive example by defining the patient's biosphere as his bed and the immediate environment of his room. A very valid goal for a person who is restricted to those confines would be to walk down the hall or wheel themselves to a recreational area. A valid goal of a person who is only able to move his arms may be to learn to transfer himself to a wheelchair. Therefore, this definition of goals defines the person's physical environment and uses mobility or some aspect of activities of daily living as life goals. While these may seem small in terms of our perception of human growth potential, they are very strong supporters of quality of life. A goal demonstrating tremendous growth potential would be the progression from wheelchair to walker or walker to cane. The goal may be being to ambulate only ten steps more a week, or the length of a hallway to a socialized dining environment.

This is only one description of growth that must define quality of life. Another description relates to those things in the creative mode, such as the ability to write poetry, paint, and become involved in other creative enterprises. The Grandma Moses concept is not limited to those people who have intrinsic creative capability. It should be described as another component of maximizing human potential, and along these lines, we must give everyone the presumptive creative ability that can be developed by proper programming in a supportive environment. To the degree that people can learn new occupations, this must be attempted also.

Another component of our definition is usefulness, which may be the development of productive work or self-care, and is intimately linked with independence, growth and self-esteem. By the same token, our final component of quality of life, self-sufficiency, while not a synonym for independence and usefulness, offers a slight variation to round out our definition of quality of life. These words are not platitudes and cannot be treated as such. They are all part of the psychosocial model implementation program, and there are reasonable measurement tools that can, if appropriately developed, fit into a very rational surveillance process. This will be discussed further in the chapter on regulatory compliance.

MANAGED ENVIRONMENT

The concept of managed environment represents a fundamentally different way to administer institutional life.

As a first step in understanding what the managed environment is all about we must return to our resident-centered management concept. What will bring about the highest quality of life for our residents? In the simplest terms, the environment must supply those things which collectively produce quality of life—and make them our institutional goals. Thus the environment must produce or encourage physical well being, independence, enhanced self-esteem, etc. Let us analyze the environment on those dimensions.

Self-Esteem/Dignity

This is a most important quality of life and one that is viewed by many as essential for longevity and happiness. Although self-esteem is an internal characteristic, it is a function primarily derived from the external world, so that the primary clues an individual has as to his/her self-value are those that are supplied by persons within the structured environment in which they live. If an elderly person is treated with dignity, that will internalize as an enhancement to his or her self-esteem. The problem that we find in imparting dignity or enhancing self-esteem is that caregivers themselves may not have these characteristics within their own personalities. In short, a caregiver who does not have his/her own self-esteem cannot effectively treat people in a dignified manner, and consequently will not encourage the development of self-esteem. Since we recognize that caregivers are the primary support system for the self-esteem of the resident, we must take the first step of enhancing the self-esteem of the caregivers.

Certainly a job, or those things that happen within the work environment cannot reverse a lifetime of societal negatives. It is well known that the workforce which gives direct hands-on care and relates most intimately with residents has, as a group, rather low self-worth quotients.

The most important first step, therefore, in this aspect of the managed environment, is to structure the work environment so as to magnify the value of the employee. This can be done in seminar form or through training. It can also be accomplished by structured reward systems (which are usually absent in the current nursing home system). Input should come from family and community members to deal with attitudinal problems of employees that often prevents proper self-esteem from developing in the residents. Enlist family and community members to support and enhance staff self-esteem.

One program that has proven successful is the bringing together of caregiver, family, resident, and administration in a learning experience where the needs and problems of all parties concerned are shared. This form of sensitization allows transmittal of positive feedback to the caregiver, and also opens a channel for caregivers to vocalize their grievances with the work environment, with family involvement, and with resident response.

When a successful interdisciplinary approach to the "welfare" of the caregiver is dealt with appropriately, the negative attitudes first observed among this group of employees changes. Several things happen. First, the positive attitude and bolstering of that individual's own self-esteem is easily and volitionally transferred to the resident. Second, because the positive attitude and self-esteem are directly related to an individual's ability to learn the technology of their job, the nurse assistant or orderly will learn technology faster, retain it longer, and implement it more effectively—all, of course, to the betterment of resident care. So this recognition that caregivers cannot enhance the self-esteem of the resident until their own self-esteem is dealt with should be a primary goal of any managed environment. This includes, as we discussed, all of the accoutrements of modern technology that can be brought to bear to make the workplace a sound and positive environment for the employee.

Another important element in bolstering self-esteem is the establishment of an organized residence council to allow participation and expression of views, to afford individuals the opportunity to show leadership; and to allow residents to gain prestige among peers. The creation of a variety of organizational entities, such as a welcoming committee, hostess committee, program committee, or menu committee all are very successful in restoring the decision making capability and leadership potential that has been lost.

Independence and Self-Sufficiency

The need for independence and self-sufficiency in long term care residents relates inversely to the phenomenon of overdependence on the institutional service. We see this syndrome develop very soon after the admission to a nursing home or intermediate care facility. This institutional dependency is a very complex process that is often resident-driven rather

than institutionally-created. As a resident comes into a protected environment, the fears of living alone are abated, and the need for basic care and
attention satisfied. As these primary needs are met by the institution there is
a reluctance on the part of the resident to give up any of his or her new
benefits. Those choices that an individual had while living in the community
are removed, especially if the institutional regimen is highly structured in
terms of, for example, bathing and eating. A combination of organizational
rigidity, and the residents' need to free themselves of worry and fear creates
an institutionally dependent individual very quickly.

The problem of how to counteract this situation is complicated by the
satisfaction that staff derives from a well-organized and tightly scheduled
delivery of services to the resident. While efficient scheduling allows any individual staff person to organize his work well, at the same time, we reduce
any personal flexibility that the resident still may have. We concurrently
eliminate one very critical factor that encourages and enhances independence: that of choice. The lack of choice in matters such as when to
take a bath, when to eat, when to get dressed or when to go to bed is a
critical institutional aspect of making a person dependent.

The issue of independence and self-sufficiency cannot be dealt with in the
resident care plan, which some experts suggest incorporate all of the non-
health components of the psychosocial system. Quite the contrary. It is the
administrator's responsibility to design flexibility into the scheduling of
staff when it comes to choices—for example, bedtimes. Entirely too much
reliance is placed on the nursing home staff for setting schedules that will
either present, or fail to present vital options to the residents. There are too
many examples of these organizational inflexibilities being designed to
benefit staff, and not the resident. It is of the utmost importance that the
administrator assume, as part of his/her responsibility, the development of
a managed environment to create this flexibility. Caregivers should also be
educated—as part of this same responsibility—in the development of their
own methods for implementing this new philosophy of a managed environment. Very often, when apprised of the importance of independence and
self-sufficiency, the caregivers themselves can design workable flexibilities
into their schedules and incorporate these successfully into their daily efforts.

The resident care plan—in terms of the resident doing as much as possible
for himself falls short because it allows an unnecessary conflict to develop
between caregiver and resident: if the caregiver does not want to do
something, for whatever reason, and can successfully list that particular
task as something that the resident himself should accomplish, the plan
itself could be utilized to the disadvantage of the resident. The responsibility
for formulating policy relating to independence and self-sufficiency is that
of the administrator and not the director of nurses. The director of nurses
may incorporate specific instructions that more closely define the degree to
which any individual resident should be self-sufficient.

Thus, it is the responsibility of the administrator to create an atmosphere
in the institutional environment that fosters this delicate process of encouragement and positive change. When caregivers understand that it is the

policy of the house, and that they will be evaluated on the basis of their understanding of and ability to implement this form of psychosocial policy, a great change comes over the working force. No longer is it governed or directed by resident care plans and individual assignments, as per tradition. It is governed instead by the mandate of the organization and its managed environment. No longer will they assume that bolstering of self-esteem and encouragement of self-sufficiency and independence are part of a job specification that is tracked by a resident care plan and monitored by a nurse. Instead, we have now created a new dimension in which the environment supports and fosters these characteristics. Caregivers are taught their personal value and shown ways to deliver the kind of supportive interpersonal communications that work on behalf of the resident. If, in fact, employees buy in to this environmental mentality and feel part of it because of their own enhanced self-esteem, the strength of the improved interpersonal bond between resident and caregiver alone will create the positive components required to make the environment work.

Independence and self-sufficiency can be augmented by properly designing the physical environment of the resident. For example, what can be more dependence-producing than the ambulatory resident finding it difficult or impossible to read room numbers or find the correct hallway, or locate the telephone. What could be easier than designing this particular environment with color combinations and lettering that remove or reduce this form of dependency? What about a reality orientation program that constantly supports the residents' understanding of his physical environment with large clocks and large calendars posted in strategic areas? What about painting the public telephone area in distinctive colors, or having signs at the intersections directing residents to the dining room, to the recreation hall, or to the back terrace?

Growth

Any discussion of growth for an institutionalized elderly resident should be consistent with the limitations inherent in a nursing home community. In its most elementary form, it should mean the opportunity to improve oneself on any level. The most immediate level would be the creative—the opportunity to learn how to paint, to write poetry and to sculpt should be made available. Intellectual growth, too, is feasible, in terms of programs in history, politics, and economics. But even more important is the understanding that growth may mean an individual's ability to achieve a goal. If we define growth in this dimension, there are a variety of options available to the resident. It may be that the goal for a particular resident is simply to be able to transfer himself out of the bed, or it may be that the goal is to walk ten feet down the hall and return to his room. In any event, goals relating to physical capabilities take primacy in our managed environment: the ability to feed, dress, to ambulate are all part of the growth potential. As we discussed before, the acceptance of personal growth as a value to be achieved will incorporate the co-operative efforts of caregiving staff and any other individuals who become a part of this managed environment.

Physical Well Being

Now we address what is ostensibly the largest component of nursing home delivery—the health component. Recognizing that the physician may spend as little as 10 minutes a month dealing with the resident, the responsibility for the health component falls on the director of nurses. The health component in our psychosocial model, however, serves only as an intervention and support for the managed environment. It is not the main consideration.

This concept fosters the belief that the administrator is responsible for the managed environment, and not the Director of Nurses, or the Medical Director. Health service, as an intervention, consists of traditional bedside nursing, augmented by rehabilitation that attempts to prevent regression, improve activities of daily living, and encourage mobility and ambulation. The responsibility, therefore, of the Director of Nurses is more particularly involved with assuring the delivery of the medical technology for which she is trained. She is also responsible for making sure that her staff understands the concept of the managed environment, that they are trained appropriately, and that they perform all the necessary requirements of the psychosocial model.

The Players in the Game

Who then is responsible for contributing to the managed environment? The easiest definable entity is the nursing service, because they are in contact with the resident more than any other group. But we define different roles for nursing: first the traditional, technically oriented delivery; then the people whose traditional obligation is augmented by taking additional responsibility for the psychosocial managed environment. However, we must include the other people who enter this environment as well, because what we are after is the development of a mosaic that includes contributions from many parts of the nursing home world. This takes into account, for instance, that the housekeeper also is a predictable part of that environment and must also buy in and be taught to communicate in an appropriate supportive manner. The food service worker, who can give so much to the appropriate serving food and contributing greatly to the ambiance we require in our food service. To the degree that family and community also play a critical role in involvement of this managed environment, they are the final pieces to the mosaic of psychosocial support that we are attempting to develop. We have defined the role of the family and the community on a different level, but here we pull them in as very important elements of positive stimulation for the environment of the resident.

From previous discussions we conclude that a major aspect of aging is a series of losses. If the administrator takes the responsibility of developing an organization whose goal is quality of life, then that organization must reinstate that which has been lost: dignity, independence, self-sufficiency, health, and self-esteem. The managed environment is the primary and most successful way to achieve these goals.

IMPLEMENTATION OF MODEL

The primary barrier to implementation of the psychosocial model is the attitudinal make-up of the people who are decision makers in the long term care system. In other words, the limitations are primarily that of accepting the concept and creatively developing methods to implement the model. When it was presented to a class of professional administrators some time ago, there was some acceptance because of the idea being perceived as a mom and apple pie situation. There was much defensiveness on the part of the medical model supporters, saying that we who run medical model facilities are very concerned about the psychological needs, and they describe social programs that they had. However, on close inspection, this is a form of defensiveness, because when asked to design the model of delivery of their own facility, very few came even close to the delivery scheme of the psychosocial model. Virtually all the students in the classes that I have taught came up with a medical model with an increased social component, which is not what we are discussing here.

Certainly the enhancement of the medical model by increasing the social component of care indicates some acceptance of the concept, and is better than no movement at all. In these schematics, however, it was still a doctor-centered service, and the augmentation of the social services essentially made a more acceptable medical model of delivery. Conceptually, however, it was the same thing. Although I take a position that attitude is the primary barrier, it is often represented as economics that is the primary barrier. The view that the only way the psychosocial model can be delivered is by substantial additional financing is not correct.

Stretch Capacity

It is my contention that a large majority of organizations have the capability to do just a little bit more with what they have through the utilization of both idle time and the generating of greater levels of performance with existing human resources. In other words, if people are properly motivated from top to bottom in an organization and buy into the concept of psychosocial managed environment with the mainstreaming concept of community involvement and the development of the family input into the care system, a higher level of performance will be achieved.

I have seen instances of facilities, who after having agreed to the merits of this concept, were able to develop a variety of programs that went a long way to achieve the goals of the psychosocial model. On many occasions it is just a creative use of existing resources that can turn the trick.

Let us discuss some examples of creative uses of existing resources. One method is that different types of staff training must take place. One very successful way is to alter the existing curriculum to emphasize the psychosocial needs of the patient and family. In my experience this emphasis on training is most effectively accomplished by bringing into the training milieu family, management, staff and resident. Under proper professional facilitation, these sensitizing training forums, if handled properly,

PSYCHOSOCIAL MODEL

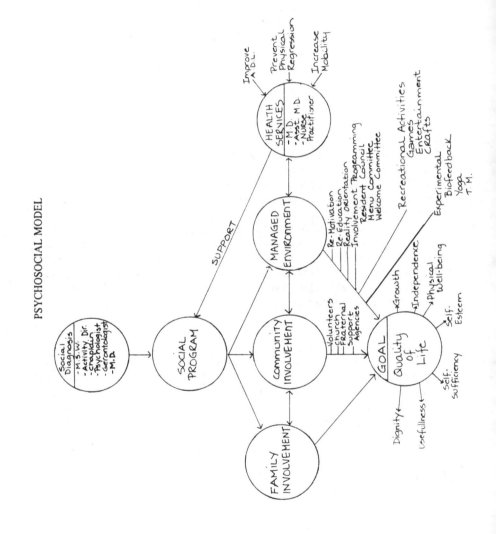

MEDICAL MODEL

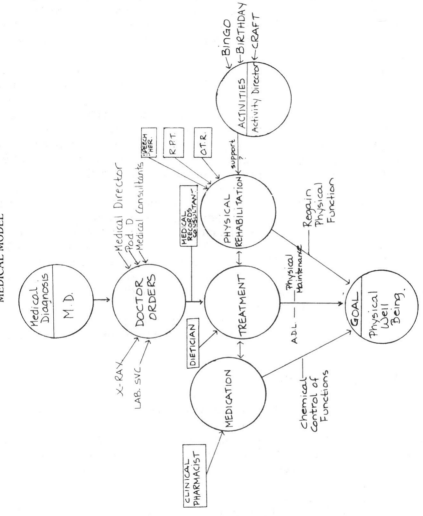

will go towards the heart of most staff training problems, which is dealing with staff attitudes and low staff self-esteem. It is my opinion that the same resources currently utilized for the training of medical technology should be reallocated for this psychosocial training. After attitudinal changes take place, then the needed technology may be taught. When this sequence of retraining occurs, the technology is learned better, applied better and retained longer. The use of training time to enhance the staffs' own self-value or self-esteem makes sense if one realizes that one cannot impart dignity or encourage self-esteem on the part of the resident if one does not have it himself.

Another very good example of using existing resources in different fashions is the redesigning of the work responsibilities of the activity director. In most facilities, this individual is responsible for direct patient services, both group and individual. If, however, this individual's time is used to mobilize community resources, such as church groups, volunteer corps, fraternal organizations, service organizations, as well as to develop family groups, major changes in the institution will take place, and the movement towards the psychosocial model will be achieved with no additional resources.

As I mentioned, attitude is the primary barrier. Certainly if one were to take the position that there is not enough money in the system to allow for the augmentation of the medical model that is needed to develop the psychosocial model, you will be stymied. Certainly the system is underfunded in many aspects. What I find, however, is the attitude that money is the only way to move toward the psychosocial model, which is a cop-out that prevents creative thinking and the utilization of existing resources in a much more successful manner.

If the definitive psychosocial model requires additional funding, then that should be explored on a different level, and become a part of public policy in long term care.

Professional Training Barrier

Next in importance to the basic attitudinal barrier that is found in getting people to accept the psychosocial model is the fact that virtually all of the professional people involved in implementing the psychosocial model are trained in the acute facility. There are very few people who are not trained in acute hospitals or acute hospital methodology. Nurses, dietitians, pharmacists, physicians and other paramedical specialists who form the core of the team find it very difficult to shake the doctor-centered model. Even social workers who have the opportunity, as part of their training, to learn more about this other mode of delivery are often coopted by the acute mentality.

The acute hospital is a service that is primary high medical technology and low psychosocial involvement. With an average length of stay of about seven days or under, how could it be otherwise? All of the training to have people function in this high technology arena must of necessity short change psychosocial training, and to a great extent the attitudinal sets that are the primary barrier to movement toward the psychosocial model are created by the intense acute medical model training needed to make that model so successful. What this means is that for the person who wishes to take the leadership of moving an organization toward the psychosocial model, he or she must initially address this barrier of the acute hospital mentality. This means that at some point a great deal of extra training must take place. This is the job for leadership as it applies to the transition from acute model to psychosocial model.

Value of the Psychosocial Model

Let us assume that the apparent value of the psychosocial model in terms of the development of a higher quality of life for the resident is reward enough for making the effort to develop it.

But let us look at some of the other aspects of the psychosocial model. First of all, there would be very clear economic savings if certain benefits of the model pays off. For example, one of the most burdensome of the services rendered in the nursing home is care of the incontinent patient. Yet many studies indicate that a high percentage of patients incontinent in nursing homes are not organically impaired, and that to some extent, incontinence is related to the psychosocial mentality of those patients. It is not hard to conceive of incontinence as a result of anger or hostility toward not just life's rewards, but to the insensitive care and negative environment the patient may be living in. There are many examples that demonstrate quite clearly that a person who has high self-esteem and has been treated with dignity, in a positive environmental atmosphere, will not want to be incontinent. This suggests that incontinence, which is a result of anger, depression and hostility is therefore not the result of organic impairment, will be reduced substantially. In facilities that have implemented the psychosocial model, we see that incontinence is a much smaller care problem with essentially the same resident population. As the care of incontinent residents decreases less resource is allocated for that very time consuming service. This lower utilization of resources can either be a money saving thing or can allow you to reallocate those saved resources for further implementation of the program.

The impact of the psychosocial model on the staff is most significant, because once one's own self-esteem and importance is established as part of a care team. When service is viewed as very meritorious and humane, there is a surprising change in work attitude that very often results in less sickness, less industrial accidents, and greater level of productivity, all of which have economic benefits for the facility.

Reduced turnover and the ultimate ability to attract a more competent person to the workforce are also side benefits of this psychosocial model.

Applicability of This Model

While we have concentrated on the implications of the psychosocial model for the skilled nursing facility, the basic tenets discussed herein relate to all the components of the continuum of care.

Correspondingly, the conflict between the acute model and the psychosocial exists in adult day health care, home health services, etc., all of which are part of the continuum. Therefore, if one accepts these basic concepts, one may be able to implement them in whatever component of the continuum he/she works in.

Future of the Psychosocial Model

To a great extent the medical model was a derivative of the thinking in the health field at the time of its origination. In much the same way the psychosocial model is an offshoot of the problems perceived in the medical model of delivery.

As our society changes with the continued development of technology and the slower development of our sociological mentality, there is every reason to believe that the psychosocial model will evolve into some other form of service delivery.

It is reasonable to assume that as the demographics of the elderly population change as well as a variety of care-oriented variables, so will the model of delivery change. Some of these variables are the change in self-perception of the newly emerging elderly and the evolution of other social factors such as the nuclear family, public policy, and changes currently taking place within the acute hospital system. These are but a few factors that will push for the development of even newer models of delivery of service for long term care that will themselves be derivatives of the newly defined psychosocial model.

The problem that we will find in this evolutionary process is that different facets of our society evolve at different paces. It is quite possible that the demands of our society for a new model will change at a speed much faster than the ability of the health system to respond to it. In essence we'll have a replication of the inability of our health delivery system to respond to the societal need for the psychosocial model.

Benefits of Psychosocial Model

A major benefit of the psychosocial model is in direct reference to the continued criticism of the delivery of skilled nursing services by the community. One of the elements of the medical model, in its ultimate analysis, is that even under the most optimal circumstances it will never respond to the total expectations of the community. The end result of the psychosocial model will. As a matter of fact, the expectations of both patient, family and community that will be met by the psychosocial model should be the primary standard of the measurement of quality of care throughout the system. To carry this one step further, it may even be advisable to substantially reduce the somewhat rigid quantitative measurements of traditional medical model delivery so that those freed up resources may be applied to the psychosocial model. We will leave this topic with the hopes that those people involved in public policy formulation will recognize the import of this concept, and develop those studies necessary to incorporate the psychosocial model in the public policy governing long term care.

Mixed Delivery Systems

While we have attempted to define in somewhat academic terms the distinction between the psychosocial model and the medical model, we must recognize the reality of the institution's functional needs.

The guidelines for Medicare prescribe that a primary function of a skilled nursing facility is to rehabilitate and discharge back into the community. And although this function, because of a variety of limitations of the systems, is usually limited to a small percent of the admittees of any particular nursing home, it does exist. That component of the operation of the skilled nursing facility that relates to an intensive rehabilitation program and discharge back into the community, would normally focus more intently on the *medical* model of delivery.

What this indicates of course is that the facility must be able to deliver both forms simultaneously. These therefore are not mutually exclusive processes, but are delivery modalities that can coexist in a managed environment. If we accept these two models of delivery as antithetical, we will not be able to do justice to the actual resident profile in the skilled nursing facilities.

Some nursing homes have up to 30% of their residents covered under the Medicare program, who are receiving intensive rehabilitative services. The nonprofit sector of the long term care system normally only has two or three percent of their total resident days in this category. Many of those resident days relate to people who will continue to live in the facility under either private pay or public assistance coverage after Medicare benefits are over. One of the phenomena that we see when an elderly person is moved into a skilled nursing facility is that in many cases their homes, i.e., apartments, hotel rooms, etc., are filled in their absence. This loss of their home creates almost impossible discharge problems when going from a skilled nursing facility back into the community as a disabled person. Landlords and neighbors, are not amenable to the variety of problems posed by disabled (even marginally disabled) elderly people who are rehabilitated after a stroke, hip fracture, or other similar problem.

Probably the best approach to dealing with the need to have some component of the skilled nursing facility focused on a short term intensive medical model approach is to augment the psychosocial model with greater rehabilitative technology. This would most likely occur in the addition of added staff time in physical therapy, occupational therapy, and comparable rehabilitation modalities. This would better approach the problem than to have a separate section in the nursing home dealing exclusively with the short term in-and-out kind of resident. It would also encourage the staff at large to be rehabilitation oriented, in those (majority) cases where there is little or no possibility of discharge back into the community.

THE PSYCHOSOCIAL MODEL:
THE NON-INSTITUTIONAL ASPECTS

Although we concentrate on the skilled nursing facility because of its predominance in the long term care system, we must also look to non-institutional delivery services to best examine the psychosocial model. Any service that must be delivered on a long time line *must* make a conscious effort to be more attentive to the psychosocial needs of the recipient. Towards these ends, the assessment tool must be carefully balanced to include both medical and psychosocial inquiries. Nothing would be worse than a home health service, or adult day care service that focuses exclusively on physical rehabilitation, and the medical needs of the recipient. By the same token, fulfilling the creative needs of the recipient of home care and adult day care, may be a vital factor in helping these individuals to cope with the many hours they frequently spend by themselves. If we visualize a fully-served home care resident receiving visits five days a week, we must also understand that those 4 to 6 hours of attentive care still leave the recipient with 18 to 20 hours of idle time per day. How constructively the recipient uses idle time may encourage wellness or create sickness. We must, therefore, be able to enhance the environment and encourage creative or constructive activities during the absence of direct hands-on treatment. One of the most challenging problems we face, in dealing with home care or adult day care, is that of creating a wellness-oriented environment that utilizes time away from direct hands-on treatment in such a manner as to be supportive, not only for the specific treatments, but to the total quality of life.

The transposition of the medical model to non-institutional services need not be made if the basic tenets of the psychosocial model are understood. The de-emphasis of the medical component and the calculated weighing of the service in favor of its psychosocial components is most important. It must be recognized for these people that the community and family component is every bit as important as for the institutionalized. The managed environment can be transposed to a person's house or apartment, so that the various daily requirements of an ambiant environment can be created in that person's own living room. Neighbors can be trained to do certain supportive tasks. Friends, relatives, community organizations and church groups can be factored in a planned and supportive way to aid the lonely, isolated, frail elderly person. This transposition of the institutional psychosocial model, if made with a great deal of integrity, can radically improve the quality of life of the non-institutionalized person.

ORGANIZATION OF
A LONG TERM CARE SYSTEM

We will now discuss long term care in a different dimension. As we recall from our review of the historical evolution of the system, there are three primary components: the nonprofit sector, the public sector, and the proprietary sector. Each one has had a significant impact at different points in history, and each has different developmental characteristics. Let us review these three systems and how they interrelate to form the entire composite.

INTERRELATIONS

While describing interrelations, we must pay some attention to the direction of these relationships and, ultimately, discuss trends and projections of the future. Suffice to say that this brief exposure to the primary components of the system does not adequately describe the interplay between them; nor does it describe the reality that integrated systems of the future will be combinations of all of these systems, or that in any one particular unit of service, several systems may exist symbiotically.

To be more explicit, there is reason to believe that the somewhat historic lines of demarcation of a profit making business and a nonprofit making business are becoming more obscure. There are examples of proprietary elements creating nonprofit spinoffs for corporate purposes, much the same as our examples of nonprofit entities having profit making components. There are situations where a nonprofit corporation will build a facility and lease it to a proprietary management group to operate. There are examples where a profit making organization will build a facility and lease it to a nonprofit organization. There are many examples in the public sector of contracting proprietary entities because the economics demand such a relationship. So as the system becomes more complicated, so does the clarity of definition of each of these primary components. Let us describe these relationships a little more explicitly by example.

It is very common for a governmental health system to contract out for services that they cannot render to profit making or nonprofit organizations. It is often more economical, and in terms of dealing with large slowly moving bureaucracies, much faster to achieve the service. Contracting out is particularly common in situations where poor planning has prevented the governmental entity from moving with enough speed to meet the demands of the community. For example, governmental entities contracting out for nursing home beds with proprietary systems when they have no capacity for home health services. By the same token, we see nonprofit organizations seeking support from governmental delivery systems and contracting out with profit making enterprises for addition of additional services.

Besides these economic arrangements of convenience, a decided competitiveness has emerged between these three systems. The competition usually evolves when a resource is short, or where the supply and demand for any particular goods or service creates market tension.

Organizational Comparisons

NONPROFIT SECTOR: REASONS FOR EXISTENCE

In the last 100 years, the primary motivation for the creation for non-profit care facilities has been the need of a particular group to take care of their own. The emergence of religious, ethnic and fraternal homes for the aged in the 1800s insured that a particular group would be able to offer their members a way to be cared for in an appropriate way. The primary force in the creation of the nonprofit homes was this parochial view of caring for "our kind of people." Expansion of the nonprofit sector with highly restrictive admission policies for specific groups became somewhat mollified in the '50s and '60s with the advent of civil rights laws and affirmative action guidelines. To some extent it was tokenism when people of different religions, races or ethnic stocks were accepted for admissions, but it did indicate a breakaway from the rigidity of these specific care organizations. Currently, nonprofit organizations are much more open in their admission practices, and the emergence of a "generic" nonprofit format became apparent in the late '60s when community groups who had no distinctive fraternal, religious or ethnic linkages formed to take advantage of the variety of benefits that nonprofit status bestowed upon the organization. The benefits of tax exemptions and other preferential treatment and government funding actually created a new rationale for creating a nonprofit organizational system. Even with these new configurations, however, there was usually a clearly defined group in mind, even though sometimes this group was defined by a tight geographical focus. Additionally, with the emergence of substantial government financial support through the Medicaid, Medicare and building construction programs, the intrinsic non-discrimination requirement of the federal government enhanced the process of open admission policies.

Because of tax relief, the nonprofit status offered relatively modest groups the ability to care for their members without the spectre of significant taxation. It also allowed charitable fund raising because donations to nonprofit organizations are tax deductible. Charitable fund raising and tax benefits allowed a greater percentage of the operating costs to be utilized for direct resident services.

Funding Sources

The majority of nonprofit organizations begin their efforts with a private funding drive. The sponsoring organization is able to gather enough money from their own reserves or from their members charitable donations to construct a facility and begin to fund the operations. Sometimes private sector (bank or government) financing is used to augment funds that come from the support group.

The funding vehicles open to nonprofit organizations include: (1) conventional mortgage loans, that is through life insurance companies, savings bank, savings and loan associations and pension funds; (2) FHA programs through the vehicle of HUD financing; and (3) the utilization of revenue bonds.

As we mentioned, the most common vehicles used to fund nonprofit development are the conventional mortgage loan, gifts, and admission/ entry or founder fees. Other sources are private placement of taxable bonds, tax exempt revenue bonds, state housing finance agencies, and public taxable bonds.

It should be remembered that financing must include equity as well as primary and secondary debt considerations, so that the combination of total financial patterns is quite varied.

In recent times, funding for these organizations has come primarily from government due to the relatively lower cost of these monies.

GOVERNING BODY STRUCTURE

The governing body of nonprofit organizations usually comes from the leadership of the sponsoring group. By the same token, new board members come from the group's constituents, and to some extent there is an element of self-perpetuation and even nepotism. For those organizations whose sponsoring group is not a clearly defined ethnic, religious or fraternal group, but community based, the governing body is usually a group of representative leaders from that community. Replacements to that governing body also come from the specific community of constituents. Normally the board is responsible to the support group for the functioning of the institution; thus, the constituents form the group most significantly involved in judging the quality of care rendered at that facility. The board of directors of a nonprofit organization have a variety of responsibilities covered by both federal and state laws that make it different from governmental or profit making organizations. There are strict conflict of interest regulations, as well as severe limitations on their involvement in political activity.

Nonprofit boards usually hire a professional executive to run the organization. The professional executive who reports to them is often linked in some manner to the basic tenets of the constituent group.

Nonprofit organizations are noted for the substantial involvement of the constituent group in the day to day operation of the organization. While this can create many administrative problems, the end result will be a more responsive, supportive community.

GOAL

An easy way to view the goal of the nonprofit facility is to subsume the goals of the constituent body. In the case of a nonprofit organization that was formed primarily to serve that constituent body we would say, at least initially, that the primary goal is enhancement of quality of life of its membership. The supposition that the members of that constituent group felt strongly enough about their collective needs to form their own non-profit entity is a strong indication that they are looking after the needs of the elderly members of their group in terms of shared values which that group holds. Communality itself may be a goal of the group: that is, bringing together elderly isolated members of its group so that they may share the aging experience in a communal way. While each of these interest groups may have different cultural, religious or ethnic values, it is safe to say that their primary purpose is to bring about an improved quality of life for their elderly members. Unfortunately, the term "quality of life" has become an undefinable buzz word used to describe almost any facet of our existence. However, in our discussion on modeling, we do establish a reasonable definition of quality of life with factors that are quantifiable.

If we assume that quality of life is the primary purpose for the formation of the nonprofit entity, it is easier to understand the operational policies and procedures and the way that the supporting bodies view both finances and the ensuing operational program. Certainly these groups do not organize and create such a facility with the intention of offering a marginal form of existence to their membership. Most of these groups wish their elderly to be cared for in a "proper" fashion, i.e., one that will afford them much more than they would be able to get living in the community at large. When a nonprofit institution is developed its function is also to represent the values of the group it represents, and to clarify its essential characteristics to the community at large. This adds an incentive for the facility to offer an environment and services that portray a strong view of that particular group's values.

OPERATIONAL FINANCES

The financing of the operations of the nonprofit long term care facility is not unlike the financing of long term care services in the other sectors. There are three primary funding sources: private payment from the recipients own financial resources, government, and organizational funding. These three sources vary in proportion to the composition of the group of individuals who utilize the service.

One of the characteristics of the nonprofit sector facilities is a tendency to serve more people in the middle and upper middle income brackets than one would expect. In facilities that have a primarily non-indigent population there is, as noted above, great emphasis on organizational funding and private payment from the recipient. With indigent populations, obviously, the government plays a greater role. We will deal with these three sub categories of funding separately.

PRIVATE FUNDING SOURCES

Individuals who are not indigent have some sort of income, either through their own direct assets, or through pensions, retirement funds, etc. These collected monies constitute the private contribution towards the operation of the facility. In most cases these are monthly rates. The management of this form of payment is usually described in detail in the admission agreement to the facility.

In some facilities where there is a large initial fee or a buy-in of some form, there are special provisions to allow the pool of the funds created by this initial buy-in to support the operations.

GOVERNMENTAL

The most common governmental source of funding is social security, which either goes directly to the facility or to the resident. Social security may in many cases be "invisible" to the organization if it goes directly to the recipient and is utilized by him as part of the monthly payment. In many cases, however, it goes directly to the institution and is augmented by whatever other sources are agreed upon. Social security plays a significant role in the determination of the Medicaid payments.

Medicaid, which is long term funding for elderly in skilled nursing facilities, establishes a liability component that requires the recipient to contribute a certain amount of their monthly income. In many cases the liability is equal to the social security check.

Medicare plays a very small role in payment for long term care services. Because of its restrictive coverage it only applies to a relatively short period of service immediately after an acute episode in a general hospital. Therefore, the nonprofit facility must not only be a skilled nursing services, but must also be approved at Medicare's level of service.

There are a variety of other sources of government payment that include Veterans Administration, railroad pension and others. For those living in federally subsidized housing, government support of "Section 8" housing allows a primary government-funded grant with a relatively small recipient contribution.

ORGANIZATIONAL FUNDING

As the percentage of residents who are funded through the public assistance programs increases, there is an anticipated increase in the funding responsibility (subvention) that comes from the organization itself. For example, in life care situations where individuals pay in front-end money, there is a presumption that these monies held in a reserve (as mentioned before) are utilized to support operations on an ongoing basis, regardless of what the monthly resident fees may be. In many situations we find that people literally run out of money, outlive their resources and find themselves covered instead by public assistance. It is a commonly accepted organizational responsibility to continue the care of these individuals to the extent agreed-upon in the admission statements. In most of these cases—income from government or the personal resources of the resident are inadequate to fund the quality of service required in the facility.

If an organization does not generate enough revenues from private pay, government sources, or intrinsic funding that comes from the organization's financial reserves, a most common phenomenon occurs. The constituency of that organization is called upon to clear any deficits incurred due to the short fall from the traditional sources of funding. For example, it is well-known that Medicaid funding is virtually subsistence level; even when utilized in a totally appropriate way, it does not afford the recipient more than a marginal existence. Most nonprofit facilities choose to offer those services that they feel appropriate for the quality of life of their constituent members and decide to fund the difference with community wide or constituent fundraisings. In some cases, this comes through annual contributions. In other cases it comes through periodic major fundraising drives to develop extraordinary reserves that will allow the facility to operate at a higher level. In many cases donations are solicited continually to support the quality-of-service needs of the facility. Requests for charitable gifts from family or friends of people seeking admission to the facility are made, in some cases, before, during or after the admission. Such practices have in recent times come under intensive scrutiny by the law. Such solicitation, therefore, should only be done within very certain, clearly defined and legal guidelines.

In some cases, such as with church sponsorship, the central church organization will fill the financial gap or underwrite the deficit caused by the disparity between normal revenue channels and actual cost. This strain on organizational resources is often the cause of serious internal problems that revolve around the merits of allocating limited organizational resources to the subvention of the operation of the long term care facility. There are ongoing dialogues with constituent contributors over the merits of these services and to the degree that this constituent concern exerts control over what may be seen as operating indulgence, idealistic goals of quality of life may be compromised.

Public Sector

If we again relate to the English poor laws of 1610 we find that the reason of the existence of the public sector facility is based in law. Being a legalistic structure, the substance that defines the responsibility of the legal jurisdiction relates to the social and cultural climate that existed at the time the law was created. Law, therefore, defines the public sector facility in terms of the secular responsibility of the government to render care and services to a defined population. The incentive for the law was the impact that the population in question had on the entire population. Since the community was beleagured by the elderly and disabled, it behooved them to create a law that made the care of these individuals the responsibility of the community as a whole. The motives, therefore, may not have been charitable as much as protective in nature. It was a way to prevent direct confrontation with these individuals within the daily structure of community life.

This method also, as we understand now, encourages removing the less healthy or able from the mainstream of a vigorous society. The reverse is noted in countries which are underdeveloped and have, in an industrial sense, not achieved the success of those in Western Europe and America. In these cases, there is still a strong emphasis on familial care of the elderly.

CAPITAL FUNDING

Being a creation of the legal system, one would correctly assume that the capital needed to construct a public sector facility also must be generated by the legal jurisdiction for which the law was created. In most cases, this comes in the form of a city or county bond that must be paid off by the city or county, and in many instances incorporates state or federal financing. Since the public sector has had virtually no growth since the 1930s, more modern methods of financing have been directed almost exclusively in the renovation and upgrading of old physical plants.

Organizational Structure

The administration of a public sector long term care facility is usually in the hands of an individual who works for the government and is part of that government's bureaucracy. Since throughout the country most state and local governments have some form of civil service, it is a correct assumption that the administrator is part of that civil service system, and must therefore report or be responsible to a component of government within that jurisdiction's governmental structure. Traditionally, city or county long term care facilities have at their helm both an elected official and an appointed official. Depending on the size of the governmental organization, the administrator will report (in the case of large jurisdictions) to a chief executive officer, or to that person's counterpart in a smaller bureaucracy. It is rare that the head of a long term care facility will report directly to an elected public official.

The sponsoring body, which is the ultimate governing body, is usually a board of elected officials. Since this governing body is a product of the political part of the governing system, the goals and objectives of the organization are strongly influenced by their political imagination. Therefore, the community's primary access to the administration of the facility is through this governing body. In most cases, however, the secondary access on an operational level is continuous and direct. The administrator of a public sector facility finds that he has many many viewpoints to contend with. The jeopardy of management in public sector organizations is considerable, and since the constituency is the community at large, opinions, views and directions are multitudinous.

In other words, the administration of a public sector entity is fraught with all the hazards that exist in any job totally open and responsive to the public.

Goals

The goals of a public sector long term care facility are spelled out in the laws that created it. Usually generic goals exist for offering humane care for those less fortunate than others in the community. Very often we also find the contradictory caveat that encourages us to also respect the drains on the taxpayers resources. At the present time funds needed to support programs at long term care facilities are in short supply. Most public sector facilities find themselves fighting in a political milieu for limited public resources. Very often the vested interest group that has a stronger political point of view gets a larger piece of the limited community resources that are derived from taxation. If we recognize that at present elderly needs are usually on the low end of anyone's priority list, we can then reach the conclusion that public sector facilities serving the elderly receive less than their fair share of monies derived from the taxpayer. In point of fact, public sector facilities throughout the country are perceived, by the community, as offering marginal, or at best merely acceptable service since the only corrective action available would cost taxpayers money.

At present, however, most public sector long term care facilities are run at taxpayer-supported deficits. When we discuss future developments, we will see how this particular form of deficit underwriting will be affected in times to come.

PROPRIETARY SECTOR

Reason for Existing

As the name *proprietary* indicates, this sector exists to make a profit on invested money. I'm not saying there are no other reasons for proprietary enterprise to begin, but its basic goal is profitability. Should there be no profitability, there would most likely be no proprietary enterprise in the LTC field. Occasionally, one hears of communities who sense the need for services to be rendered to the elderly members of their population, but find that the only way these services can be rendered is to invite a proprietary organization to deliver the services. In these cases, we see a unique combination of public sector and profit making enterprise. This combination will be discussed later but bears a critical examination in light of the dynamic changes currently happening in the system. The fact that profitability exists at all as a motive in this field has been challenged for many years. A more thorough discussion of this will take place in the chapter on Ethics.

We must, however, be cautious not to exclude any motives other than profitability because that, too, would be a misconception. Giving the proprietary sector their just due, we must credit them with acknowledging the rendering of human service as their actual reason for existing.

Capital Funding

Proprietary endeavors are usually funded initially by contributed capital from owners. This investment capital is usually augmented by back loans or in the case of privately funded housing, loans from federal government in housing and urban development. In the early stages of development of the nursing home system, with the large numbers of sole proprietorships, we found would-be owners collateralizing their home, taking out personal loans, and gathering up funds from family contributors. As we are now in a system that is moving towards corporate control, much more sophisticated methods of funding exist, including using float capital, acquired from refinancing existing building stock and money pulled in through stock acquisitions. The value of this capital in the open market is productivity-based (a standard for the total economic productivity of the profit making institution) meaning the capital invested in the profit making facility must produce what it could produce in the open markets or more.

Since this method of private funding allows for maximum leverage through the process of second and third mortgages on any physical plant, it was possible to develop proprietary enterprises where there was very little capital actually invested. This very thin method of financing was also very risky, because of the multiple notes on any property. Repayment demands had to be generated from operating expenses which left the ownership with minimal operating funds if the real estate indebtedness was to be paid off. Therefore, this form of financing, although profitable in many ways, created at its inception a heavy load for the operating budget to bear, and has contributed, to some extent, to the marginal service level offered by many of these facilities.

Organizational Structure

Proprietary long term care facilities are administered by a salaried administrator who usually reports to the ownership or its representative. Since these organizatons are closed corporations, the ownership is usually a partnership or corporate board. Although there are still many owner-administrators, the numbers are rapidly thinning because of the growth of corporate ownership. Another characteristic of the corporate ownership structure is that with size comes the development of regional management units that fall between the administrator and the actual corporate decision makers. So on one end of the spectrum an administrator may report to the ownership (either a partnership or small corporation) consisting of only several people, and on the other hand, he may report to a regional officer or manager who in turn reports to the corporate head management, which in turn reports to the corporate board. The corporate ownership pattern, which follows the development of multicorps in non-health fields, implies also that the proprietary long term may represent only one segment of corporate activities. The conglomerate could be producing tires, importing raw materials or any of the multitudinous activities in which large corporations are often involved. It is quite possible for the administrator in a nursing home to find his policies developed from a corporate headquarters primarily involved in another field of activity. This remoteness separates corporate decision-makers from the frontline administrator in an unhealthy way.

The corporation may be insulated and isolated from that which occurs in the field, while a sole proprietor, who is on the premises, may be much more sensitive to the events in the nursing home. Under these circumstances, corporate leadership would not respond, for example, to community input which is so vitally needed to achieve true quality of resident care in these institutions.

Goals

Consistent with its reason for existing, the primary goal of a proprietary facility is to make money in one form or another. Certainly the profitability factor as a primary goal does not exclude quality of life concerns, nor does it necessarily mandate poor quality, negligence, or any other dark prospectus. Profitability has been managed in many cases while quality is still quite clearly evident. We must recognize that if we view the full spectrum of proprietary endeavors in the long term care field we will see many examples where quality of life is quite high.

The misuse of the profitability motive, however, has been a public concern for some time, and this ostensible problem will be discussed later under the chapter on ethics.

Profitability can come from many different directions. The most obvious is profit from operating income. But the most common is the profitability inherent in the ownership of the real estate. The tax advantage and ability to re-finance are but two of the components of profitability that has attracted hundreds of millions of dollars into the profit making sector.

Fiscal Underwriting

While profitability from operating is a primary goal of administration, the organization must at least break even on operating income and expense. Many factors come into play which reduce profitability such as a low census; too low private pay census; and poorly controlled expenditures. There is the possibility that the proprietary facility will run a deficit. In any long time line a facility that consistently loses money is either reorganized to a level of profitability or disposed of or closed. It is only on rare occasions when a losing business operation is continued, and that is usually for certain tax advantages.

If an ongoing deficit *is* incurred, one of the most common moves to balance income and expenses is a service reduction. As a matter of fact very often a service reduction is mandated if the required degree of profitability is not met. For example, if the standard return in a particular proprietary facility is to produce $100 per month per bed, and in order to do this services must be compromised significantly, then that will be the administrative imperative.

In many cases, there may even be situations where the profitability factor is not met at all and radical changes in the service are therefore required. Occasionally, a corporation that does not have a profitable investment will invest more money in it to upgrade the quality of service in the hope of attracting a higher percentage of private paying residents. So we now begin to recognize that the mix of residents in any facility is critical in determining the economic viability of that facility, as well as the service level that is possible given organizational goals and objectives. It is rare, however, to find a proprietary organization that will bolster the quality of care in a deficit-run organization.

INTERRELATIONS

Now that we have described the three major sectors, we should readdress the high degree of interrelationship between these sectors.

As we have noted in the past, there was no relationship between the three. We now find, however, interesting combinations of nonprofit, public and proprietary working in combinations that offer the population at risk appropriate services.

Some of these examples are as follows:

The public sector may contract to the proprietary sector: A governmental entity not wishing to create capital intensive services may contract out to profit-making services specific functions, such as rehabilitation care for psychiatric cases, or for the developmentally disabled. Once these services are rendered elsewhere, however, the guidelines of the sponsoring body may or may not be adhered to. It is part of the challenge, when a public sector entity contracts out to a profit making entity, to maintain the required standards of the public sector.

Another very common combination is the relationship between a proprietary management company and a non profit sponsor. For example, a non-profit sponsor could build senior housing, and yet contract out for a proprietary firm to handle management. Another possibility is a profit making construction corporation owning and operating the physical plant but contracting the actual operations to a non-profit entity.

The ability of the proprietary sector to go from the beginning of an idea to the implementation phase in a very very short period of time has proved of tremendous value to the public sector interests when a particular crisis has emerged. The proprietary sector's ability to decide quickly, gather capital quickly, and go into the implementation phase very rapidly has made it an invaluable resource for a community faced with a significant health crisis. At least, this holds true in the field of aging and long term care. The proprietary sectors' ability to move capital through bureaucracies with a clean, although opportunistic motive of profitability, has saved the day in many cases.

The ability of a non-profit group that could not possibly raise construction capital to lease a physical plant owned by a profit making company has allowed many non profits to flourish.

Since the public sector's primary responsibility is for the care of the indigent population, it has allowed the proprietary systems to serve the more affluent component of the system while the tax supported public sector cares for the less affluent or indigent part of the society.

What we have seen additionally is the emergence of non-profit organizations that do not have a specific constituency, but that are created primarily for the tax shelters offered the constituent investors. In these cases, non-profit status and the proprietary mentality may be indistinguishable.

Our review indicates the multiplicity of many non-institutional services, and social dynamics forcing the creation of services in areas that do not have the capability of capital formulation. Inevitably, private money shifts into these areas. It is already happening and appears to be a major direction for the future, that is, the dominance of private capital in the non-institutional sector of the long term care continuum.

Management Information Systems

The current revolutionary stage in communication technology is characterized by an increasing emphasis on the utilization of information. The development of electronic data processing technology has enabled organizations to compile and effectively access more information than at any time in the past. This "information revolution" has become indispensable in modern management. Applied to the long term care organization, it is a tool for effective decision making and fiscal control. Computerization has become a necessity not a luxury; every long term care organization should maximize this tool to the fullest advantage.

As would be expected, the industrial sector of our society has taken the leadership in this technological rush. The health component, which is the country's second largest industry, lags significantly behind. Within the health field, the long term care system lags considerably behind the hospital system, so that what we are describing here is the beginning of the technological restructuring of an already frail and unsophisticated system.

True to the historical relationship between the acute system and the long term care system, the long term care system is modeling itself on the acute system, with certain exceptions. For one: as the new technology came on the market, it was assumed that long term care delivery units, being relatively uncomplicated, did not lend themselves to the direct automation enhancements which seemed natural for acute hospitals. As a matter of fact, the small size of skilled nursing facilities appeared to work against maximizing automation and support manual internal management systems.

We must develop a new concept of the already-oversimplified management technology that currently governs the administration of long term care services. Our new concept must emphasize speed and budgetary savings and be able to highlight the value of new management information as it relates to decision making, problem solving and the reduction of productivity bottlenecks. A total system would provide hospital staff with benefits such as extensive query capability, electronic mail and message switching, file sharing, electronic file storage, and data base research for management and health professionals. And a well-planned internal network would link workstations with a central system, giving the hospital staff the opportunity to create, merge, modify and redistribute the appropriate resident and cost information.

This same idea could link the long term care service with a larger external network. The incorporation of automation on a large scale in a small organization may create a situation of resource shifting rather than economic savings per se. In general the automation of routine employee function usually frees up those employees for the performance of tasks previously excluded because of time constraints. As we view larger long term care services with many units of employees, it becomes theoretically possible to reduce the number of employees with the aid of automated systems, and therefore to reduce corresponding units of cost. Not so with the smaller facility. While the cost saving factor usually is found to be primary in the minds of most managers, the value of cost saving in small operational units must be looked at differently. Certainly, if any automated practice would cut down on one or two hours of your key office manager's work or reduce the need for outside consulting services, that would clearly demonstrate a cost saving. But let's look at the advantages from a different viewpoint.

While we are continually using the skilled nursing facility as the more complex organization in the long term care continuum, each of those service elements within the continuum, to different degrees, could use some form of automated function. Extending ourself beyond individual service units within a continuum would be the ability to track residents' movement between services and have the ability to collect data from a variety of points. This is especially true when the long term care provider is part of a community organization. Think of the variety of services inherent in these support organizations. The automating of the interactions between various components of the continuum of care itself creates a system that becomes integrated of necessity. This systems approach will be referenced when we deal with future trends and should be reflective of the augmentation of the long term care system as a whole.

In determining and assessing appropriate technology in the long term care delivery unit, our first step is a comprehensive needs analysis, which should be completed before moving into any automated system. These needs will change as the service becomes more automated. That is because different combination of uses for your automated equipment will become more apparent.

Let us assume that long term care automation needs can be broken down into the following sub-systems:

One would be a patient diagnosis and treatment system that includes information derived from such hospital departments as laboratories, pathology, EKG, radiology, pharmacy, rehab and nursing services. *Two*, a patient record system, which would involve medical records, admission and a financial eligibility program. *Three*, patient appointment scheduling and an order system which would include all patient care departments and support services. *Four*, patient accounting system which involves cost center analysis, receivable accounting and credit and collection functions. This would also include patient trust information, a billing system for a variety of payors, and a payable component that allows the hospital to pay its bills. *Five*, an expenditure and general accounting system which includes budget, payroll, materials management systems, in addition to gathering charges for resident services. *Six*, the personnel system. *Seven*, general supportive services including industrial engineering, and preventive maintenance. And *eight*, a management control system, which effectively links the entire structure together.

As you go through the needs assessment process there is always the question of what is a true "need." These questions might be resolved by considering such factors as fundamental as facility size. With larger organizations, automated offices that take advantage of word processing, electronic messaging, scheduling, etc., would be most effective. Smaller facilities, on the other hand, might want to focus more on an integrated business function system, which would automate several basic facility departments at one time. An objective analysis of the service is the best insurance to guarantee that the system selected is one which is the most appropriate, useful and cost-effective. These decisions, which include a comparative study of comparable services should be augmented by a third party opinion. This third party will provide the degree of objectivity necessary to select the option most appropriate for the particular service. It is a rare administrator who can produce a thorough needs analysis without assistance from a third party, most usually a system consultant who has a broader or different view of the hospital's function. Since computer sales firms claim to offer a panacea to all management needs or problems, I would suggest viewing the needs analysis on several levels.

REPLACEMENT OF FUNCTIONS

If replacement of functions will cause a reduction in your operating costs equal to or better than the costs of the automation, it is a positive indicator. This type of cost benefit analysis will usually include costs relative to the implementation, such as salaries for system analysts and data processing personnel; file preparation; and testing costs. In addition, there are costs associated with application software. These may involve system maintenance and enhancement; additional hardware; vendor staff costs and employee training. Finally, timing should be considered to estimate the approximate period of planned payouts; the expected dates of system implementation; and return on investment.

REVENUE PRODUCTION OR COST AVOIDANCE

The needs analysis may determine if the automated function will produce net revenues or avoid future costs in amounts equal to those incurred while converting. Automation for other purposes is an add-on expense, unless proven otherwise. Automation that simply creates idle time or greater ease of tasks is hard to justify. Automation that creates greater degrees of accuracy, where these degrees of accuracy are important, is a value.

SOME KEY VARIABLES

Size of the facility may be considered to be the first variable. Sheer volume of information needs will help to dictate the type of hardware to be procured, and indicate if the facility is conducive to automation at any level. Small facilities, although lacking the volume of information needs found in larger organizations, will still utilize many of the fundamental business functions considered to be compatible with an automated system. Large facilities, on the other hand, often present different problems in the sense that each major department or business function may have specialized needs and require its own dedicated system. In either event, the system should be designed so that eventual total organizational integration will be possible. Integration should not be compromised by the size of the facility.

Another variable to consider is whether the facility is a distinct part facility or is a freestanding facility. The distinct part must interface with other components of the organization. The freestanding facility may discover information needs which are so specific to that particular facility that they may be non conducive to total automation. The many possibilities that exist for automation might well be reviewed by an objective external industry consultant.

Character of ownership must also be considered when performing a comprehensive needs analysis. When the facility is owned and managed by a private sector for profit corporation, decisions involving the investment of time and money to facilitate automation must be made by the corporate leadership. It may well be the case that private sector long term care administrators will be required by the corporation to implement a comprehensive management information system, in as cost-effective a manner as possible. The needs analysis in this situation may have been performed by corporate representatives, and cost factors are likely to be viewed in relation to the total corporate plan.

It may also be the case that functions involving reimbursement might be considered as a higher priority for automation than functions which do not directly relate to fiscal enhancement. The administrator in this case finds himself in the position of mediator. The main task would be to prove to corporate representatives that information needs will be met more adequately with these non-fiscal enhancements.

Public sector administrators may experience a very different scenario. The public administrator might be much more involved with the role as the facility representative who is charged with the task of objectively examining the organization for the good of the public and to protect the public investment of time and money. In this regard, constraints on budget expenditures may be more stringent than in the private sector. The administrator should be prepared to explain large fiscal outlays, and expect that a certain amount of budget reduction will occur because of political pressure placed on the budget review process.

The final factor to be considered is the relationship of a facility to other corporate units. It may often be the case that an automated system must be developed and constructed to interface with various components of the corporate structure. In particular, is the provision of accurate and consistent financial reporting. Certainly, the performance of the facility (and of the administrator) will be monitored in terms of the amount of profit produced, and the degree to which losses are minimized. Perhaps the needs analysis might be geared toward interfacing with an existing corporate system to insure the success of information transmittal.

Comprehensive planning, therefore, is the key to successful assessment of the organization's potential for automation. Automation itself has become a necessity if the facility is to compete in an expanding marketplace.

In completing our needs analysis, a basic guideline might be that all functions not related to direct resident care be automated. The needs analysis process must be seen as ongoing, and involving a long term expenditure of time, money and human energy. The risk of not attaining high return on this investment appears minimized if the process is approached in a prudent fashion. The rewards might be the development of a facility which will function well in the economic environment of the future.

Assuming that our attitudes towards automation are positive, systems applications and issues regarding implementation may now be further examined.

The long term care administrator finds himself faced with a bewildering array of computer hardware. Selection of hardware, relating to a comprehensive needs analysis, involves the comparison of mainframe, mini, or microcomputers. The needs analysis should have indicated the type of computer appropriate for the size of the facility. A mainframe computer is enough to process the data needs of several organizations. A minicomputer will serve a large size (250 beds) adequately. The average sized skilled nursing facility of 100 beds or less, would use a microcomputer with tailored applications software. These computers are generally fast and relatively inexpensive.

It is possible to timeshare with other organizations on one central mainframe, but difficulties such as response lag time and inflexibility in meeting the facility's specific software needs are considerations that contribute to the negative appraisal of long term applications of mainframes. The minicomputer tends to be a more flexible type of machine, with the capability to tailor its functions to the information needs of specific facilities. The minicomputer, because it is installed at the facility, allows for a considerable amount of internal management control and monitoring. This on-site location of the hardware also permits an increased emphasis on data security. With on site location the administrator can be sure that sensitive financial data or the residents' medical information is not leaving the premises. The minicomputer, however, because it *is* located at the facility still represents a substantial initial investment of funds. In addition to actual hardware costs and costs for ancillary devices known as peripherals, the physical environment for the computer ideally needs to be specifically constructed. Microcomputers are designed to be "user friendly" and generally are quite compatible with most physical environments without construction of special rooms. Service contracts for new computer equipment usually guarantee that the organization will not exprience excessive downtime due to hardware malfunction. In the contemporary competitive computer market, most manufacturers are interested in developing good client relationships, and will generally be co-operative in the servicing of these accounts.

The microcomputer application, although greatly publicized, may have specific limitations in the development of a comprehensive integrated network for long term care facilities. Although the microcomputer is user friendly and relatively inexpensive, it is generally very specified in terms of its application. Because of its reliance on soft or floppy disks for the program, it is generally not capable of running more than one type of program at any given time. The microcomputer can't handle a large data base and there is often difficulty in having different brands of machines communicate with each other. The microcomputer is sufficient for the specialized needs of specific departments, but may be inadequate if it is envisioned ⁺o be the cornerstone of a comprehensive integrated data network. The recommendation would then be to investigate the use of the minicomputer, and, once committed, to obtain the best service agreement possible with the manufacturer and their company representative.

Once the computer is procured, the task then becomes one of obtaining the most appropriate and cost effective programming or application software. Although specific applications to the long term care environment will be discussed later in the chapter, there are some considerations which require immediate decisions. This involves the issue of whether to develop application software in-house or at the data site, or whether to buy a package developed by an external software company. It should be noted that the purchase or lease decision applies also to computer hardware, and the completed cost benefit analysis will be the guide as to the viability of either fiscal option. Also, in terms of software, contracting with an external data processing company or service bureau is also a possibility. Service bureaus are companies which are able to provide a wide variety of data processing functions with their own equipment for a negotiated fee. An important decision will be whether or not to work with an in-house programming staff and computer system, or a service bureau, in order to obtain the desired results and staff expertise. Making this decision will involve an in-depth evaluation of the software package to determine whether it meets the institution's objectives and whether it will be worth the extent of organizational change required to implement the system. Flexibility and capability to respond to in-house needs and priorities is usually more easily obtained through an in-house service. An in-house service, under the management control of the institution, does not have to conform to standardized requirements which service bureaus impose on its subscribers. Institutional management also has the advantage of easy access to local personnel for consultation, and the ability to make the quickest possible response to required change.

Very often the most critical decision faced by the administrator will be whether to buy or lease the new computer system. Lease contracts are variable and change from company to company. The most sound course of action is to have the lease agreement reviewed by your attorney to guarantee that the contract may be terminated if services prove to be unsatisfactory.

In this case the financial risk is minimized. There are some basic guidelines that will assure you of reducing the risk in system purchases: first, be sure that you know who is responsible for what—is it you or the vendor? The second, is to have an organized way to confirm what you are getting—do a detailed analysis of the contract and its relationship to your needs analysis. Third, be sure all transactions are on paper, signed and handled in an appropriate legal manner. Fourth, remember all standard forms can be changed and amended and may have to be altered to protect your interest as a buyer. You should recognize that contract and purchase agreements have a degree of complexity that may call for scrutiny beyond the traditional legal review. It would be well worth the money spent to call in a legal specialist who can evaluate and advise on the numerous subtleties inherent in this transaction.

THE SYSTEM COMPONENT

If it is decided to have an automated system within the long term care service, a functional organizational analysis must be completed using, if possible, a technique of structured analysis and design. A structured analysis involves charting the flow of information through the organization by means of a pictorial diagram. This diagram delineates data input into the system, major business functions, data transformation points, and various defined data bases. The graph presents an easily understood schematic for a potentially complicated system. Using this diagram, system users can actually visualize the present system, make modifications in it, and eventually diagram the ideal proposed system. This analysis serves the dual purpose of providing programmers with a specified structural format from which to design software programs, while at the same allowing system users to define in detail the functions of their work area. In this fashion, an organizational and technical analysis is performed in one operation.

One crucial variable in the successful implementation of an automated system in the facility is the attitude of the computer users, who are primarily the employee group. The inclusion of "the user group" in the design and system analysis of the plan is vitally important and will lay the groundwork for a positive attitudinal base. Fear and anxiety are often the result of a computer's installation, due to their reputation for displacing individuals or for placing them in work environments for which they are not prepared. This fear and anxiety may translate into resistance to the system or, in the worst case, outright damage and sabotage to the computer, software, or implementation program. Incorporation of user input, allaying of job-oriented fears, and the eliciting of user co-operation in the total program are imperative to assure a successful implementation and facilitation of the goals of the system.

The plan, therefore, should be to involve the users from the beginning in the design and implementation of the computer system. An atmosphere will develop whereby they feel they have a personal stake in the system because it ultimately will make their work more efficient and effective.

A last factor to consider in the system design and implementation is the location of equipment and the ergonomic issues of man/machine interactions. The long term care facility presents specific problems in this context because of noise reduction needs and the space restrictions that normally exist. For example, there should be a distinction between workstations for employees who use them full time versus those who only use them occasionally. Space for computer use should be designed prior to installation. If not, the use of the area likely will be cluttered and ultimately decrease productivity. In a nursing home, the best place for a terminal is at either end of the nurses' station. This reduces traffic through the station to get to the terminals and minimizes disruption. Terminals should be away from the main trafficked areas around nurses' stations or from a similar functional area in other long term care services, so that the key people can concentrate on their work at the VDTs (video display terminals). The screens should be positioned so that visitors and residents cannot read confidential information on the screen while standing near them. Alcoves near, rather than in, workstations are best for noisy printers. They are then accessible but do not disturb staff and residents.

Proper lighting to avoid eyestrain from glare on the VDT screen should be coupled with specially designed glare shields which are currently available. Indirect lighting bounced off another surface such as a wall or ceiling is best for VDT operators. Windows can also relieve eyestrain allowing operators to change their field of vision for relaxation. The height of the tables and chairs and the angle between the operator's eyes and the screen are all factors that are critical to the long term comfort and work effectiveness of the people using the equipment. Literature on the appropriate alignment of chair, desk and VDT is readily available.

FUNCTIONAL AND DEPARTMENTAL APPLICATIONS

Proper flow of information is the thread that binds the separate, yet interrelated, departments or functions of a long term care service. Top management performs the function of linking all the component parts together (in a management sense) to insure that these parts perform their tasks now and in the future. The system should allow the information gathered from divergent sources to be combined into formats which are easily understood and directly applicable to management functions. It should also have the flexibility to be used by all levels of management.

It is beyond the scope of this text to explore further the issues of appropriate transferral of information, reformulation and sharing of new data, choice of specific technology for the construction of an accessible data base, etc. Needless to say, the utilitarian value of an accessible data base will be most significant in the future operation of long term care services.

AUTOMATION AND STRATEGIC PLANNING

As we will discuss under the chapter *"Planning,"* short range, intermediate range, and long range planning for the long term care service must be an ongoing function. The computer allows us to store and interrelate information for financial and policy modeling, utilization, legislation and a host of other variables. It reduces the risk that important data will be overlooked or insufficiently factored in. The long term care administrator must be able to justify decisions regarding equipment acquisition, expansion, policy changes, etc., to an ever larger and more vocal public. No longer are these decisions and their impact restricted to the governing body. The fact that government, insurance carriers and various other elements in our society are now involved in the health/human service complex means that accuracy of factual support for decisions and plans is no longer a luxury.

RISK MANAGEMENT

Administrators also are faced with greater degrees of scrutiny of safety and resident care procedures than ever before. This translates into an increased incidence of liability claims. An automated system designed to coordinate incident reporting and prevention is a realistic component of the overall service. The fact that problems are easy to record, analyze, report and track will hopefully expedite the development of preventive measures.

PUBLIC RELATIONS

There are many examples of the application of computer automation to track fund solicitation, volunteer activity, board functions, public relations, correspondence and communication. Certainly anything that can improve the image of the facility or service in the eyes of the community would be considered valuable, since often the long term care organization's ability to function at all is a matter of community support and receptivity.

COMPREHENSIVE FINANCIAL INFORMATION SYSTEM

Financial management is intimately related to both fiscal and non-fiscal data elements. The reality of the 1980s revolve around increasing efforts by government and private industry alike to reduce healthcare expenditures at a time when an improved medical technology and an aging population creates an increased demand for healthcare services. Thus, cost reduction and containment are daily facts of life to the administrator. Activities involving cost containment, reduction, and rationalization of expenditure can only be successful by relying on an automated system to deal with the vast array of information needed for the decision making process. The analysis of financial alternatives will require extensive modeling and forecasting capability, on which to base decisions affecting the service's competitive position in the marketplace.

The administrator of a long term care facility will be responsible for finding programs that maintain and extract the maximum detail, or else that have the capability to expand to the needed level of detail for future use. For example, a nursing home may require a very flexible chart of accounts with the ability to do simultaneous reclassification in terms of additional criteria that may be demanded by third party payors. Audit trails should be as complete as possible, referring to the offsetting accounts used for posting of transactions, as well as containing adequate descriptions for each leg of the transaction. Financial statements, in a variety of configurations, should be available on demand, complete with budget, prior period, and per resident comparisons. Accounts payable should have the ability to automatically distribute expenses according to the mandates of the government or governing body. This system should have the capability to monitor purchasing activity in detail by vendor, item or general ledger account number. The ability to budget by item is also desirable, as is the ability to instantly see exactly what you have purchased from a vendor or quantity of the item to date. Accounts receivable should be as fully automated as possible, with direct and easily auditable tie-ins with resident census, and all billing sources, rates, resident movement, and other appropriate detail. Payroll is a logical function, as is an employee data base. The system should be able to automatically calculate and distribute employee benefit costs. Patient assessment programs should also be able to calculate the nursing needs of each unit in a skilled nursing facility, or project a variety of staffing pattern needs in any long term care activity.

Each of the previous systems that we have discussed should have user-definable formats for forms and reports. These forms and reports should be modifiable at the user level to the greatest extent possible, and screen inquiry capabilities should be extensive. Finally, the system should be able to check data for errors before and after entry.

RESIDENT INFORMATION SYSTEM

At the core of any automated information system is that collection of data relating to the resident. The primary input source of resident demographic information is the admission system. This system should have the ability to adequately generate pre-admission reports and to maintain a referral monitoring system for future admissions. The system should also have the capability of capturing resident data up front to provide for accurate reimbursement information. Daily census reports, transfers and discharge information reports should also be generated. To be effective, this system should be integrated so that all of the functions we have described will be accessible to users. Data retrieval and modification, then, is a primary concern for the resident information system which is more immediately linked to the medical records system than other functional services within the long term care agency. In these records reside the total history of a particular resident or service recipient. In addition to upgrading of pertinent resident demographic information, the medical record should be designed to monitor chart deficiencies and routine clinical information. In an institutional setting, the system must also provide for an adequate system of location and control of charts. Efforts should be taken to protect the confidentiality and safety of medical records from individuals unauthorized to view such information.

In short, the system will attempt to improve the tracking of record locations, to minimize manual work involved in medical records, and to provide overall faster service to the users of these records.

SECURITY ISSUES

Because information concerning residents is usually accessible in a medical records system, the security of this confidential data base becomes a major consideration. The proliferation of computer terminals throughout a facility or service unit represents the possibility of inappropriate access. In addition to the resident information, financial and accounting information must also be protected. Protection of information means adequate controls. Although passwords and log-on codes offer a certain level of security, there are currently more sophisticated measures such as fingerprint recognition, magnetic card access, palm geometry, and time locks that restrict access to the terminal or to specific levels of information. It is important to recognize that security has become a specialized field, and it would be most appropriate to have a consultant refine the security of your system to a satisfactory level.

UTILIZATION REVIEW

Since some form of utilization review is prevalent in all areas of long term care, the automated system is ideal for supplying the supportive information upon which to make many judgments, define classifications, and analyze levels of care. Patient care profiles and their relationship to levels of care designation within any long term care service serves as a valuable monitoring device for resource utilization and allocation. It is possible to track physician utilization patterns and to isolate individual physicians who may be contributing to financial losses for the facility due to inappropriate requests for services. This relationship between technology and the production of information has had a significant impact on the practice of medicine. Those monitoring systems that relate to clinical practice must be developed with the cooperation and collaboration of the medical practitioners working with the long term care service.

NURSING SERVICE

In a skilled nursing facility the nursing department may represent the work area where the greatest percentage of hands-on resident care occurs. Because of this proximity to the resident, the nurse represents the best source of data gathering due to their extensive observation of the resident. There is a definite trend to develop a nursing information system that can tie into the facility-wide information system and link to the overall resident care information program. It is quite possible that nursing care systems will represent the major thrust of patient care information systems over the next five to ten years. It is clear, also, that since all data about the patient is located at the patient's bedside the new focus of such nursing care systems will be at the bedside where care is given and data generated. A great deal of effort will be applied to the development of bedside information systems in the next five years.

Additional to the bedside system concept would be the inclusion in the system of order entry and results reports to and from every ancillary department. The nursing station can then serve as an automated center for the transmission and receipt of this data, as well as all data relating to staffing resources and the quality of care.

The quality of care tools relate to six basic objectives: (1) the plan of care that is formulated; (2) the physical needs of the resident; (3) the non-physical needs of the resident; (4) the achievement of nursing objectives; (5) analysis of unit procedures that routinely are monitored and evaluated; (6) the provision of nursing care as it is augmented by administrative services. Daily staffing recommendations resulting from resident classification will allow nursing administration to change staff on individual units and to fine-tune staffing in relationship to overall resident needs.

QUALITY ASSURANCE

The direct input of resident care variables can produce quantitative documentation and summary reports normally found in a quality assurance program. The effectiveness of the quality assurance program can best be determined by the decisions, changes and improvements that result from the deliberations of the quality assurance committee. Unlimited combinations and correlations of data can be utilized to respond to isolated interests or resident care concerns. An interactive system capability allows the quality assurance department to have online access and programming capabilities. This allows for the examination of multiple configurations of data rather than the review of isolated incidents in situations. It also improves the timeliness of data and enhances the responsiveness to specific data requests.

AUTOMATION IN SPECIFIC SUPPORT AREAS

Nursing Pharmacy

Along with the departments that are directly responsible for hands on care are the ancillary services which provide crucial support. Automation is particularly adaptable to pharmacy requirements (usually found only in larger SNFs). In addition to a catalogue of various medications and chemical components, pharmacy management systems should be able to maintain an ongoing file of resident medication utilization and a schedule of prescriptions. A good pharmacy system should have a mechanism that prevents inappropriate medications from being issued, and one that highlights negative drug interactions or side effects. This function is crucial from the standpoint of control. The system should have files on both the unit doses for residents as well as the method of drug administration. A record of medications not administered to residents could be held on line and be easily accessible to pharmacy personnel. A compatibility check of drug mixtures is a function present in pharmacy system software and represents a convenient checklist for possible adverse reactions to combination medications.

In summary, the following are the key points in a nursing pharmacy safeware system: (1) the ability to interface with the facility's system; (2) inventory control; (3) drug, IV and allergy reaction monitoring; (4) 24 hour a day, 7 day a week system support; (5) clinical capability to be used for diagnostic evaluations; (6) the ability to expand for future enhancements; and (7) hardware integration within the facility's system.

The pharmacy system should also be able to perform routine functions, such as admission, discharge and transfers, profile maintenance and labeling.

Laboratory and X-ray Services

Although most skilled nursing facilities contract for laboratory and x-ray services, there would be an expected utilization of clinical lab and x-ray information as part of the overall information system. Since long term care facilities rarely have their own clinical lab or x-ray services, the incorporation of this outside information into the internal system makes the system an important tool to monitor the performance of the contract services.

Dietary System

The dietary department also presents considerable potential for system automation. The continual analysis of food service information and the extensive planning required to control these variables present clear opportunities for a dietary management information system. Although this is a relatively new software application, all indications are that it will be an important area of development. Nutritional analysis, recipe analysis and cost and budget analysis are the three main features of a dietary system. In more specific terms the system could include food intake assessments, daily recommended dietary allowances, estimated safe and adequate range comparisons by age, sex, height, weight, and activity level. It could also include nutrient analysis, virtually unlimited recipe storage, ingredient substitution, conversions and recipe variations. It should be able to produce a dietetic analysis for a resident within five to ten minutes and thereby increases the efficiency of existing staff.

Materials Management

Materials management is a sub-system that will have a great deal of value for all service components in the long term care continuum. After dealing with the initial computerization of inventory information which will include, among other things, units of measurement, date of last activity, cost of last activity, quantities on hand and inventory par level system, you can then incorporate a purveyor or vendor file which tells you whom you have ordered from, what their prices were and a variety of other vendor information. The system would incorporate purchase orders as well as disbursements, receipts, and other adjustments to inventory. It would include a direct relationship to the facility's fiscal system, including payables and receivables. Bar-coded inventory control mechanisms will be the basis upon which the system will develop, and a variety of inventory reports will be produced to allow purchasing forecasts to link into the total financial and budgetary system. The outcome will be better utilization of resources by means of tighter control of usage and lower inventory levels.

Personnel Functions

Use of automated systems in personnel management is already old hat, although in long term care most personnel systems are manual. The maintenance of personnel benefit records, insurance, liability usage, are basic functions of any long term care facility. The production of checks and appropriate tax documents are but a few of the routine uses of the automated system. For larger facilities or service systems, personnel allocation can be done in a very detailed manner allowing us to cost out specific functions much more accurately. Scheduling is another part of the personnel and payroll function that can be automated in long term care.

The future of automation in long term care is as limitless as the technology that is being developed to meet the changing needs in our society today. Ultimately we will see an integration of telephone and video communication systems in combinations not even contemplated at this time for the health field. Automation is a key to effective decision-making through the use of accurate, reliable and well-understood information about residents and about the institution's operations. Probably the most important aspect of the automation of long term care is that it requires planning and self-education on the part of the administrator. Management must understand the current system and must take the responsibility for moving it into the future. Self-education about the computer marketplace and the system options available is now required for successful management and will be the path to successful career development.

Marketing Long Term
and Senior Care Services

In discussing the issue of marketing of long term care service, we must come to grips with certain realizations about our own administrative practices.

First of all, we must recognize that the concept of marketing in our field is relatively new. As a matter of fact, it's been only in the last few years that marketing in the hospital field has assumed the stature of having specialists act as head of marketing or director of a marketing department. It is not that long ago that many far-thinking academic institutions began to teach health marketing with, of course, the emphasis on the acute hospital. In order for us to begin a serious dialogue on the issue of marketing in long term care, one must accept that marketing is here to stay and that the factors that have created the need for marketing in most of the health fields relate directly to our long term care services.

I have heard on many occasions that people have trouble with the word marketing because of its relationship to the shabbier side of the corporate world, to advertising agencies that have very low degrees of credibility, and to shabby practices in retail trade. Maybe what we're talking about is the need to utilize a different word to sooth our sensitivities. Regardless of what word we call the action, the process of marketing has a significant role in the successful functioning of all long term care facilities and services.

To carry these introductory comments on marketing one step further, we must also acknowledge that there is a wide diversity in the long term care field, and that certain elements within long term care are already on the path of developing very sophisticated marketing approaches. This will lead us into a much more specific discussion of long term care and its varied elements.

DEFINITION OF MARKETING

We should recognize that in nonprofit circles the term marketing has certain negative connotations. It is linked with "Madison Avenue" advertising and some of the less desirable parts of the retail trade business. We've also already recognized that marketing as a specialty field is relatively new in the health field in general, and it is still having difficulty being accepted as part of the acute hospital modus operandi. Needless to say, whatever we have learned about marketing in the health field has come from our experiences in the acute hospital, and that in itself must point to the need to modify practices to suit the long term care.

We must recognize that long term care is considerably different than the acute hospital field, and therefore, while certain basic techniques might be applicable, possibly definitions and processes may be quite different. One way to define marketing is a way of doing business or a way of thinking about management. Some have even called it management philosophy. It is important to spend some time in pursuing this definition of marketing because it may be necessary to custom tailor this definition to suit the long term care field.

We would have to agree that the long term care delivery unit, whether it be a nursing home, residential care facility, or adult day health, has a service that it wishes to deliver to some component of the community. The second realization that we must accept is that in order to make this linkage we have to describe the service in the most optimal manner possible to suit the perceived needs of the people that would use the service. The next most logical component of this definition is that we should be very, very clear on who the individuals or groups are that would benefit from the use of this service. We must be very specific in defining that group, and we must be very direct in bringing the description of our services to that group in the most appropriate and successful manner.

This attempt at definition of marketing falls short in that it is a brief synopsis of the marketing process. If one were to accept the premise that marketing is a component of management that assures the appropriate match between the service and the user of the service, and that this broad view allows the process to go on indefinitely, one can incorporate marketing as a bonafide philosophy of management. Once marketing is accepted at this level and incorporated as part of management activity on a routine basis, then the definition of marketing is complete. If we look, however, at marketing as a project that must take place at only certain periods of time, it ceases to become defined as management philosophy and assumes a much less significant role in the efforts of any organization to render its service successfully to a defined community. In other words, this definition of marketing is: the effort of bringing your services, which are presumably the right services to the right user at the right time, at the right place, at the right price; and that if this is your intention as an organization, marketing must be an ongoing function. So by description we have defined what marketing is in long term care.

In order to place marketing at the proper level in management process, one must note the difference between marketing, advertising, promotion and public relations. If one were to accept marketing as the "umbrella" philosophy, then these other terms would easily fit as sub-components to the broad marketing philosophy that management could choose to adhere to.

While we must remember that marketing *is not and should not be an at-*

tempt to force customers to accept a service they don't need, it may be necessary to define in the marketing approach, goods or services that may or should be needed by the potential customer. Once you cross the line, however, and attempt through marketing methods to coerce the acquisition of the goods or services by a customer, you have, in essence, crossed the line into that area of marketing that has caused great public disfavor. You should recognize that you are entering an area that *no longer is appropriate*, in my opinion, in terms of ethical conduct for the long term care field. Unfortunately, there are elements within the health system that have chosen this most negative of the "Madison Avenue" approaches to selling their services, and as a result the legitimacy of the concepts of marketing are constantly being challenged.

A component of the explosion in the elderly population is the recognition by manufacturing and retail enterprises of the enormous potential purchasing power that the elderly have. Because of the methods of marketing clothing, liquor, recreation, etc., we must be doubly cautious that our conceptual base for marketing the long term care services is not treated by the elderly population or the community at large in the same fashion as marketing a product is. This is a difficult line to walk and relates to my previous comment about defining the marketing process out of the traditional Madison Avenue definition. We are already seeing in the market place forms of media advertisement by respectable community organizations which would have been unacceptable just a few years ago. It is important during this new "free for all" that is being created by the emergence of the health field into traditional marketing practices that the marketing of long term care facilities and services is not denigrated by the more traditional practices.

To further utilize these marketing concepts, we must be able to define the new marketplace in relationship to the competitive system that is evolving. We must be able to know and understand the idea of vertical integration, the impact of hospitals into the long term care market scene and the relationship of HMOs and PCOs to this marketplace.

Before we involve ourselves with specific marketing approaches that relate to different elements within the continuum of care, I wish to recommend that the history of long term care and the chapter on the continuum of care be reviewed, in order to put the contents of this chapter in a clearer context. We must recognize that a successful marketing program can only be achieved if you fully understand the relationship of the continuum of care, and the historical perspective of long term care, to the delivery and acceptance of the services that you wish to market.

In order for us to be thorough in our exploration of marketing for long term care, we must therefore go into a thorough analysis of its elements. Let us define a marketing program in the five major steps: organizational buy-in, user needs analysis, marketing plan, marketing communication, evaluation and change.

In order for us to be thorough in our exploration of the marketing for long term care, we must therefore go into a thorough analysis of the elements of marketing. Let us define a marketing program in five major steps.

1. Organizational "Buy-In"
2. User Needs Analysis
3. Marketing Plan
4. Marketing Communication
5. Evaluation and Change

ORGANIZATIONAL BUY-IN

The most important and leading component of the marketing program is the organizational "buy-in." I am using this phraseology to indicate that the decision making component of the organization, whether it's the administration, the ownership or a non-profit board of directors, must, after careful analysis of the circumstances and need for marketing, accept a marketing program as a major organizational philosophy. If there is no organizational "buy-in," the other aspects of the marketing program will not be effectively implemented.

Sometimes, in order to get involved with the organizational "buy-in," a presentation by an outside professional through the office of the administrator may be necessary. There may be a need for a tremendous selling job describing all of the ramifications of the marketing program to the board of directors or the ownership. (Or until the administration actually says, "Yes, we want a marketing program.")

There are many deterrents to this organizational "buy-in." One of them is the fact that many long-term care facilities find that their services are in demand and that this "fat cat" status, i.e., with a waiting list for their services, causes them to wonder at the need for marketing. What must be pointed out is how quickly the marketplace changes. There are many examples of organizations that find themselves with waiting lists one day, and because of organizational or demographic changes, with low census or low utilization of services the next day.

In these cases, the marketing plan must be presented as a way to hedge against the future and protect the organization from being hit by some unknown downside risk that is hidden in the marketplace. But let's not deal too much longer with the "fat cats" who have tremendous demand for their services. Let us assume that they will be wise enough to recognize the risk inherent in complacency. Let's deal with those services that must be presented to a consumer in a competitive marketplace. Let us assume that it is important for the service to sell itself in order for it to be utilized and that the demand for it may or may not be there. Let's accept also, that there is no overwhelming utilization of this service.

It is this type of organization, where the "buy-in" has the most significance. There may still be a need for an outside individual, a specialist in marketing, to present this for acceptance by the board or ownership.

USER NEEDS ANALYSIS

After the organizational buy-in, the next most important step is to analyze the needs of the potential users of services. In the case of long term care which is a marketplace of elderly people, research must take place that will help pinpoint what the elderly need or want. Whether you start out determining the need to build a nursing home, or start a senior nutrition site, an in depth analysis of the potential customers of this service must be made. Although it may seem crass to call the elderly who use the service "customers," from the standpoint of marketing, they are people who will purchase goods and services.

One aspect of analyzing the marketplace for the elderly is to know about existing resources that have done needs analysis of the elderly population in a particular area. One resource, of course, is your Area Agency on Aging (AAA). The second is the existing local planning agency. Very often, the state department on aging or various advocate groups in the area have done their own needs analysis, and with a high degree of accuracy, can pinpoint the potential market in that particular aging community.

Additionally, there are many government publications including the White House Conference documentation, and information from the National Institute on Aging that can give you broad directions and trends that may be taking place in the marketplace. Research papers that examine the personal characteristics, habits, shopping behavior, and leisure time activities of consumers have been published in well known professional journals.

To analyze the marketplace for nursing home beds, for example, one would research out the bed quotas through the local health planning agency. A discussion with discharge planners will tell you very quickly about the demand for beds. The same process would assist you in determining the need for residential care beds. Let us assume that you have analyzed the marketplace, and determined that there is a need for a service you are currently delivering. You now want to assure yourself of a continuing, steady flow of business. This means that your marketing plan must, as we have discussed in the past, be on an ongoing program, one that keeps you in touch with the particular market of users for your service.

A most important point is that you will need very specific data. For example, it is very important to know the discharge pattern of your local hospitals to determine the referral pattern and potential attrition into your facility. It is very important to understand the nature of the continuum of care, so that you can project the potential users of residential care based on the marketplace for senior housing and seniors living in their homes. It is necessary to determine the specific number of people who are unable to leave their home for meals. This will allow you to determine if your own home meal program will have enough business to be viable. The specificity in terms of numbers of users, their geographic dispersal, and their economic capability must be done in as an exact manner as possible.

The analysis of the user market may take a significant investment and it may be worth it. It is one thing to analyze a market for a particular service that needs only flexible resources, such as additional units of personnel; it is another thing to analyze a market that will require millions of dollars worth of capital investment. Point in fact, if this is the case, and millions of dollars of capital investment is going to be required, it is to your decided advantage to have the marketplace analyzed professionally. The high degree of accuracy that a professional market feasibility can provide you, may save many improperly invested dollars, may redirect your development, or may even encourage you to cancel the project entirely.

MARKETING PLAN

The marketing plan is nothing more than a series of decisions set on a certain time scale, that will ultimately reach a certain goal. The goal in this case is the acquisition of your service by the customer or consumer. This plan will take the data received by the user research, move into the development phase so that the service is created by your organization, communicate the existence of this service to the market, and then evaluate the reception of this service by the marketplace. This plan, sometimes called the strategic plan, is worth a great deal of your time and effort, because if it is successful, you and your organization will be successful also.

MARKETING COMMUNICATION

At first blush the elements of marketing communication may appear to be very familiar. In organizational life, we have all experienced the need to produce a brochure or some descriptive literature about our service. Most likely you have gone through the process of evaluating a variety of kinds of advertisements that would be put in either the yellow pages or pieces of literature that are circulated throughout the community. Few administrative people have not been involved in some kind of marketing communication. Most of the time, however, we called it public relations and attribute other motives to this particular action. One aspect of this generic form of communication is that it probably is a public relations vehicle and should be considered as such. Not that marketing is qualitatively different from public relations at every interface; it's that public relations and marketing should be viewed as different processes to deal with different managerial philosophies. That's not to say that a particular piece of literature or action would not be both a public relations vehicle and a marketing vehicle.

Let us say, however, that we have a communication in mind that recognizes a marketing approach that requires a great deal of analysis, both from the standpoint of the specific public to be reached and the specific definition of the product or service to present to them. We then must design a communication vehicle that has as much technological analysis, targeting, and design that we can build into it.

Let us outline a few of the most common, and I may add reliable communication devices.

A. Personal Communication

In my experience, one of the most successful means of marketing communication is the individual approach, which says that you as an administrator or an appropriate member of your organization must make direct contact with the population to be marketed. If you have pinpointed a specific elderly group, or if your marketing target is for example for discharge planners or physicians, nothing is better than a very positive, well-constructed, personal appearance.

If you are in the process of marketing your nursing home, few things can beat your meeting the physician that will ultimately refer a patient to you. If you rely heavily on discharge planners, your personal contact with them is very important; let them see you and the quality of management you represent. The presumption is that you have the intrinsic capability to do these presentations. Do not overestimate your capability; if you are strong in many aspects of management, but not in this one, do not do yourself a disservice; use someone else in your organization who is better able to appeal on a personal level. The ability to communicate to individuals or groups and market directly in this fashion usually will lead to successful accomplishment of your marketing goals. To some degree, it offers you speedy feedback as to the success of your ability or to the positive reception of your communication.

Usually, however, it is best to carry with you certain written materials to leave with the people you have spoken to.

B. Printed Material

The development of pamphlets, brochures and other written promotional material is an art form unto itself. The quality, style and design vary widely, depending on the amount of money you're putting into it, the image you want to portray, and the kind of technical assistance you use in developing it. It is important that an individual who uses the personal communication vehicle, use written literature to leave or distribute. There are many professional people who can assist you in designing literature about your service. Your best approach, of course, is to get pieces of literature that can be both hand carried and delivered through the mail. Very often, pieces of distributable literature will have components allowing the user of the service to respond back to you either in a request for further information, or in response to certain questions posed in the literature. In any event, one or more pieces of printed material are imperative in virtually any marketing program.

C. Media Communications

Developing part of your marketing program using media such as radio, TV, or the newspapers, is considered by many to be a cost effective approach. The drawbacks are your lack of ability to do target marketing, and the assumption that the general public who will read or hear or see this form of communication will be self-selective. Both television and radio have free public service announcements (PSA), which should not be overlooked by nonprofit organizations. Most organizations are able to make a list of named individuals in radio and television stations as well as the key person in your newspapers who will handle news releases and public service announcements. If you are unfamiliar with how to write a public service announcement or tape one, a brief meeting with any of the PSA directors in your local tv or radio stations will clear this up very quickly. There are also many professionals in the field who can assist you in making PSAs.

In terms of using the "mass" media for marketing communication, we must recognize that there is a substantial expense, and a very difficult time monitoring the return. Paid advertising in newspapers, tv and radio are perceived to be very efficient and acceptable marketing approaches.

The yellow pages of your telephone directory are a must for any of the services that you will be selling. Believe it or not, people will go to the telephone book before they will approach information and referral agencies and other more sophisticated approaches to routing individuals into your service system.

D. Group Events

To some extent this approach is related to the personal communication.

In essence you are inviting a group to an event that could be a talk, a discussion, a multi-media presentation, a contest such as a raffle.

When planning the "event" approach to marketing, you must: (1) include developed, selected guest lists, (2) manage the logistics, (3) plan the presentations that will be made and (4) find some way to assess the success of the event.

EVALUATION AND CHANGE

The most overlooked component of a marketing plan is that which evaluates the effectiveness of your program. Monitoring the purchase or acquisition of the services you are offering is important. You find a way to analyze the reception in the marketplace in such a manner that corrective action can be taken on at least two levels. First of all, you want to find out from your evaluation process whether the product or service you are marketing has merit, and meets the needs of the consumer. The second component of your evaluation is the determination of how successful your marketing plan is: that is has your communication been successful, did you analyze the consumer market adequately, did you design and package your service appropriately?

An otherwise successful service delivery system fails because they don't know what went wrong. It could be any of one of a number of things, including misdirected mail, improper demographic data, wrong analysis of consumer economics. Very often, the analysis of a marketing program allowing you to change "midstream" may be the only thing that will save an otherwise good project. Your evaluation may also indicate that you should scrub the whole program, thus enabling you to cut your losses.

ORGANIZATIONAL MOTIVATION

It is important to understand the motivation that drives a marketing program. It should be linked, of course, to the nature of the organization and the goals that the organization defines for itself. For example, if the organization is proprietary, it can be assumed that the goal is a return on investment, or profitability. Therefore, with this in mind, the marketing approach is to develop those products and services that have a profitability factor. It should be noted that in the senior health system, there are many services that do not have an intrinsic profitability factor, and while the trend toward higher levels of income among our elderly population continue, it must be recognized at the outset that profitable versus unprofitable service options must be understood thoroughly. It is possible that, as part of a marketing strategy, an unprofitable service will be packaged with a profitable one. If the organization is nonprofit and strictly service-oriented (either a private nonprofit organization or a public sector organization) the intrinsic profitability of any service takes on a new dimension. For example, surplus revenues would be used in a nonprofit organization to underwrite or deficit-finance those senior services that do not have an economic base. Thus we see the marketing approach shift significantly between proprietary and nonprofit modes, each having its own set of values and validity, and each viewing the senior health system from a slightly different angle.

Let's now describe the acute hospital's emergence in delivering health services to the elderly. We are constantly made aware of the large number of excess hospital beds throughout the country. As part of the acute hospitals' attempt to stabilize their budgets, fill empty beds, and thus capture additional revenues, they will convert excess bed space to those services that can be utilized by seniors, primarily skilled nursing or intermediate care. Even the swing bed concept can be utilized for long-term institutional care. In the utilization of empty beds in acute hospitals, marketing mechanisms must be used that defines their activities as responding to deficiencies in the service system or as an effort to improve the overall quality of care in the system. Many hospitals are moving towards what is commonly called vertical integration. This is the purchase or control of services that relate to a form of continuity of care developed for discharged patients, such as homecare or skilled nursing services. These vertically integrated services usually keep the particular patient in a "loop" much the same as the process that takes place in a health maintenance organization. Once the patient is in this loop, the variety of services controlled by the acute hospital are marketed as part of the total package. The efforts of the hospital to vertically integrate its service is, in my opinion, primarily directed towards the economic benefits of controlling the patient as they move through different levels of services. The choice, from the marketing standpoint, has been to either market the total package of services, or to market them individually. In those cases where services in a vertically-integrated or closed system are being marketed, we must focus on the point where the patient, or recipient of service, is presented with a new service option.

When an elderly patient in an acute hospital is assessed and directed to another service, the marketing for that service should take place at that point. The discharge planner or individuals involved with the discharge, should direct and "sell" the services that would be appropriate from the standpoint of continuity of care. These services, of course, will be the ones that are operated by the hospital. The ethical problem is that, at the point an elderly person is to be discharged to another service, she is not in a position to critically judge recommendations made by the discharge planner. Marketing of services offered in a vertically integrated system (or a controlled system, similar to a health maintenance organization) must be done in a most judicious manner; reflecting on the elderly citizen's right to choose. Does this work in practice? It is difficult, at these points, to offer options of comparable services when one of these options is owned and/or controlled by the discharging source. Again, an ethical analysis of discharge practices *should* occur at these points in vertically integrated systems. An ethical marketing program will allow the senior real options to choose from. The difficulty in making choices at the point of discharge is obvious, when the discharge planner, or other individuals connected with arranging the discharge, have a vested interest in the facility-owned service. Does this vested interest allow the senior to get genuinely appropriate options in choosing his own discharge site? Or does this marketing approach arbitrarily *prevent* a person from receiving what might be the most appropriate services?

It behooves the management of these systems to understand the nature of the communication that takes place at this point of discharge and do what is both proper and ethical for the benefit of senior dischargees.

COMPETITIVE ENVIRONMENTS

The health system has not learned a great deal from private enterprise when it comes to competition. Time and again, health organizations throw themselves blindly into the competitive arena without doing the basic moves that are routine to any sensible private enterprise. Most administrators have grown up in a health arena of expanded services and mushrooming operational revenues. Because competition is so new to the health field, few management personnel are trained properly for it. Secondly, the recognition of competition by health field administrators as a big game, in which revenues are created and vacant beds filled, has rarely taken into account the possibility of failure and the consequences and impact that this has for an organization.

Marketing, therefore, must address not only the somewhat conventional approaches, but the reality that most of the people in the field are not attuned professionally, experientially or educationally to the sharp edge of a truly competitive marketplace. What this means is that many errors of omission may take place. One of the most common is overlooking the lack of demand for any given service system. Because demands for health services have historically been high, there has not really been a need to analyze the competitive positions of other hospitals or service centers. I have seen many occasions where services were created and marketed only to find that the numbers of comparable services in the marketplace prevented any one of them from having an adequate share of the market to fund their venture. It is very important, obviously, to assess the strengths and weaknesses of known competition, and spend a reasonable amount of time developing a strategy that, not only reaches the consumer of service, but addresses the existence of competition as well. It is one thing to sell a product, it is a totally different thing to sell the product in a glutted market.

The competition must be analyzed both individually and collectively. Their sphere of influence, quality of offered service and constituency must be key factors. It is important to know their economic viability to determine whether they will truly be able to deliver what they promise. It is also important to know if there are people who have shared loyalties, since we all know that people that work in health systems may often be serving several masters in the marketplace. Once we have understood our competition, we can then refine our marketing approach to truly compete.

It is very important that a marketing plan have a fall-back position that recognizes the possibility of failure. The fall-back positions must be analyzed, therefore, in terms of modifying or closing off the service. The economic impact of the services' failure must be known in advance. Nothing is worse than the ripple effect of a failed new program. The reason that this failure is magnified, is that often the new program has been designed in the first place to stabilize or enhance a wobbly fiscal structure.

During any marketing plan one must explore the regulatory paradigms setoff for that particular service. I have seen situations where an entire program was developed and marketed, only to have certification denied at a later date due to a regulatory limitation that had not been noted before. We must accept the reality that the health system, senior programs included, is controlled to the extent that regulations play an important part in the marketing plan—if for no other reason than to assure that your proposals will have the necessary government sanctions.

The competitive marketplace we have been describing, therefore, has at least two unique characteristics. One is a marketplace defined by integrated service systems that reduce the consumers' freedom of choice. In these systems price of service is most significant because the payor has the authority to limit its selection of the beneficiary to cost-effective providers. Therefore, payors can encourage the development of lower-cost providers because of the limitations of access stated in beneficiaries plans.

In short, the provider that wishes to enter the marketplace for services that are primarily controlled by payors must consider price as the most significant variable in determining success.

Secondly, for services that are selected on the basis of consumer choice, there are many variables and price is not necessarily the sole controlling factor. In this case, the payor does not have as strong a position. The consumer, who has greater freedom of choice, will factor in location, convenience and the subtleties of quality. Therefore, it is very important for the provider of service who is developing a market plan to ascertain which services the consumer will choose volitionally, as against the percentage of recipients who will be in a tightly-controlled system where most of the decisions are created by the payor. To extend this a little further: it is becoming a common practice for the provider of service not to market the consumer, but to market an intermediary. The intermediary, of course, will contract with the provider of service, usually because of the price factors alone, rather than the quality of components of the service. However, the provider of service who uses price as his only guide and marketing device is very short sighted. In the long haul, price will be only one of a variety of factors that allow a service to maintain a contract with an intermediary.

One consequence, I may add, of marketing a service solely on the basis of price, is that the regulatory standards and/or perceived standards from the consumers' viewpoint may not be met. If, in fact, an elevation of service levels must be made in mid-contract, the economic adjustment may be more than the service can bear. It is, therefore, important at the outset to market not only on the basis of price, but on the basis of long-term cost, factoring in quality, consumer needs, and professional standards at every step of the way. Although intermediaries who are buyers of health care may initially respond only to price, they themselves will learn that for long-term success they must demand a quality product, and that price alone may have a detrimental effect on their total operation.

As less and less choice is offered the consumer it can be anticipated that the process of restricted selection will result in services which are produced solely because of their economic liability. It can also be assumed that as price dominates the competitive arena, and cost shifts to less restrictive environments, numerous services needed by the elderly population will simply not be rendered, unless there exists a means for deficit financing of these services. Therefore, it is quite clear that the competitive marketplace will cream off the more fiscally viable services and leave those needed services which do not have a sound fiscal base, to either be paid for out of the pockets of the elderly or to be subvented in some manner by the public sector. Although it is not in the purview of this book, it would be important to analyze the impact of shifting economically-unsound service programs to the public sector. If these services are not picked up by the public sector and cannot be afforded by the individual elderly consumer, they will, most likely, not be rendered at all, unless underwritten by private, nonprofit entities.

Most likely, we will find several years down the road, that needed services which are not offered, will negatively impact the health of our elderly population.

The quality of life led by the elderly who have health problems can be greatly enhanced by their receiving appropriate services at the right time.

The ability of service providers to understand this dynamic and respond accordingly can be greatly enhanced by adopting a management philosophy that incorporates professional, ethical and effective marketing programs.

Advocacy

The primary advocates for people being served in the long term care system are the management and staff of that service. Unfortunately, because of the historical development of the senior advocacy movement, the primary advocates have become the adversaries.

In the early 1970s the advocacy movement grew because of major problems in the delivery of quality of care in the emerging nursing home industry. Advocacy groups took two primary directions: one was to challenge quality of care problems within nursing homes, on many levels; and secondly, to assume the role of the conscience of the legislature and community. Senior advocate groups have had some success in pricking the conscience of society. They have been able to let legislators know that the elderly do not stand alone in their fight for equitable treatment in our society. While some of the elements of improved service that has been manifested in the last few years can be attributed to the advocacy movement, much is left undone.

The three approaches that advocacy has followed have been citizen organizations, governmentally sponsored ombudsman programs and professional associations.

OMBUDSMAN

The ombudsman program initiated by the Administration on Aging in the early '70s has the greatest potential for dealing appropriately with the myriad of problems incurred in delivering institutional services to the elderly. In the literal sense, the ombudsman is a neutral person between the citizenry and the government. As it is used in the nursing home world, the ombudsman is part of an organized program that assumes the responsibility of informally conciliating grievances that arise out of resident care in skilled nursing facilities. Recently, the ombudsman program has expanded in its scope of responsibility to health-related facilities. The ombudsman programs differ considerably by locale. The mentality of the leadership and the statutory direction have often directed the ombudsman into an "enforcement" track similar to, or as an augmentation to, existing licensure and civil enforcement vehicles. In more mature ombudsman programs, the enforcement approach has been found to be very costly in terms of time and money and, in the end has failed to meet the needs of the elderly citizen. The most successful ombudsman programs are those that have been able to break down communication barriers between consumer, institution, and government, and bring to bear a rational, professional, problem solving approach to the institutional conflicts that arise. The successful ombudsman is trained to investigate complaints, to bring parties together, and to develop problem solving approaches to conflict situations. The successful ombudsman not only represents residents, but very well may represent the institution against adverse government activity, or the institution against inappropriate family involvement. No one challenges the ombudsman role as an advocate for the resident, but very often the process used by the ombudsman causes a great deal of concern and in and of itself creates the barrier for the successful implementation of the ombudsman role.

If viewed as a minisystem, the nursing home, government and community (family or consumer service) is the triangle which must be managed properly by the ombudsman. Fact finding must be appropriately conducted. Problem solving and conflict resolution must be professionally handled. Most ombudsmen are not professionals in the sense of degreed or licensed individuals, but are citizens with good intent and well-trained skills. Many people feel that the ombudsman program has been the only rational controlling mechanism for abuses that once dominated the long term care field. As the field expands in its complexity and diversity of services, the ombudsman's role will no doubt be called into play in these new non-institutional areas.

CITIZEN ADVOCATES

Throughout the country there are a variety of groups that have as their main reason for existing, supporting the rights of the elderly, and are thus named the advocates of the elderly. They have been the primary source of support and representation of the elderly to the legislative bodies that have created public policy, and have joined together with national agencies and professional associations to form a bulwark of support for the frail elderly. Their impact on the institutional sector, which was the primary reason for their creation in the first place, has been successful. Their efforts have been mostly directed to augmenting and intensifying the regulatory process. The concern many have is that they have dealt primarily, if not exclusively, with reducing negatives or protecting the down side risk of the institutionalized elderly, and have not addressed enhancing the quality of life within the facility or creating positive programming or attitudes. Many people even challenge the success of the intense regulatory policies they have helped initiate.

Because of this form of advocacy, several things have happened. One, the primary advocates, which is the administration and staff of the service, have been construed and constructed as adversaries and they themselves have unfortunately accepted this as a self-perception. The second failing of the advocacy system has been to force individual nursing homes into becoming armed camps with a variety of legalistic and attitudinal barriers to the efforts of the "advocate" groups. This problem has caused more problems than the intensified regulations have solved.

The challenge of the advocacy movement is to reconceptualize its purpose and methods of operation. The challenge of the public policy makers is to recognize that if the administration and staff of any delivery system for the elderly were to recognize and accept the responsibility of being advocates for those in their charge, the system as a whole would be further on its way to both acceptance in the community and, more importantly, the ability to deliver a high level of care to its elderly residents.

As a textbook instructing administrators in the administrative function, the definition of this advocacy role has to be more than a mild platitude. We have discussed, in the chapter of ethical considerations the problems that this mode of expression creates.

PROFESSIONAL ADVOCACY GROUPS

There are many national associations whose reason for existence is to be the spokesman for the rights of the elderly or a certain section of the elderly population. Such organizations, such as the American Society on Aging and American Association of Homes for the Aging are composed of either professionals or professionals representing institutions. As we have discussed in our public policy section, these professional advocacy groups, which some consider reflect only interests and viewpoints of their vested interest constituency, usually will join forces with the consumer advocacy groups in efforts to achieve legislative or regulatory benefits for the elderly population.

While these organizations collectively constitute the strongest voice for elderly needs in the public policy arena, they have been criticized for being self-serving and not being truly representative of the grass roots elderly whom they purport to represent. The prevalent criticism that professional advocates are essentially in business to create work for themselves is a cynical description of many worthy organizations who have contributed greatly to the benefit of the elderly population.

THE ADMINISTRATOR AS AN ADVOCATE

A properly trained administrator is the strongest and most important advocate for the residents in a skilled nursing facility or other elderly service. As discussed under the chapter of ethical considerations, very often the administrator is a double agent.

Because of this double agent status, he is beholden ethically both to the corporate values for which he works, and to professional and community values as advocate for the elderly. While the issue of proprietary enterprise in the health field is no longer an ethical one, certain components of proprietary service implementation must be challenged.

One of the most glaring aspects that creates a conflict of interest to an administrator, who must be the advocate of the resident, is the current method of compensation administrators receive when they run nursing homes. That is the *bonus factor*. There are no successful methods to monitor and assure that the lure of the bonus structure to increase the administrator's compensation will not create a conflict of interest that subverts and suborns his primary role as an advocate for the residents in his charge. It is my position that the bonus incentive in the management of skilled nursing facilities should be eliminated, that adequate salaries and benefits be paid, and that this substantial inducement to a conflict of interest that exists in the administrator's worklife be removed.

We have pointed out one critical area of the double agent conflict that could be rectified to allow the administrator to emerge as the primary advocate. The administrator must create a working environment that itself supports advocacy, by the word and deed of its staff. In order to encourage this posture, the advocacy movement must see the phenomena that I described as the "armed camp mentality," for what it is, and take a course of action that reduces or eliminates this adversary relationship with the skilled nursing facility, a relationship both artificial and detrimental to the elderly receiving care.

Ethics

ETHICAL CONSIDERATIONS

In order for me to address ethical considerations in a text on long term care, I must of necessity reduce this vast subject to something appropriate for our field of endeavor. This means that the traditional foci of medical or bioethics may be of lesser concern than those issues that are of a more immediate nature to the administrator of a long term care facility, and as such we may find ourselves defining ethical conduct in circumstances not addressed before.

The main problem, therefore, is that we will be somewhat parochial in delineating those specific areas that may relate to administrative function on the pragmatic level of those that have chosen to be administrators in this field.

The challenge is to contract normally extensive ethical discourse to the tight focus of day-to-day operations. Of necessity we must bring in personal ethics, societal ethics, and professional ethics in some combination that will give the administrator some understanding of how these components of such a vast subject impact him in his daily work.

There is also an interesting interplay between ethics, public policy and our efforts as administrators to make patient-oriented decisions.

We will discuss ethics in its broadest applicable sense and then narrow the focus of our discussion until we end up with the subject of personal ethics as it relates to the professional function. In our discussion of ethics we find an obvious conflict in ethical standards between segments of our society, between people of different cultural, ethnic or racial backgrounds, and even in the comparison of medical ethics and business ethics. What is more probable is that we will note many situations where something may not be unethical per se, but will pose an ethical dilemma. As we discuss a variety of ethical dilemmas the long term care administrator must address, we will constantly juxtapose the primary ethical responsibility over the administrative responsibility when it is apparent that they are not synonymous.

With this commentary, let us begin our discussion with a textbook definition of ethics and then define a series of circumstances that create ethical dilemmas that relate to this definition.

DEFINITIONS

As good a starting point as any are the primary and secondary definitions of ethics found in Webster's dictionary, i.e., "the discipline dealing with what is good and bad and moral duty and of obligation.'' Second, is "the theory or system of moral values" and last is "the principles of conduct governing an individual or group.''

Extending this to Peter Drucker's concept of the ethics of responsibility, I would consider the basic responsibility of an administrator to be the Biblical precept "do unto others as you would have them do unto you." Accepting this would counteract the operational distance most administrative decision makers have from the variety of ethical problems that develop in their facility. What we are defining here, then, is a priority of responsibilities for the administrator that says his ethical responsibility supercedes his job or managerial responsibility. Can we accept this premise? Can an ethical responsibility be placed at a higher level? Will it allow a subordinate administrative function to take place? Will it conflict with traditional management practices? Will it subvert as it relates to the administrative responsibility, traditional definitions of ethics?

All of these ideas are different facets of the same subject which move us to the next level of definition. This juxtaposes ethical conduct at the level of the society with ethical conduct of the individual in his workplace.

THE BUCK STOPS HERE . . .

Because of the nature of the system, the long term care administrator has the primary control over the quality of care of the service that his organization provides. A logical extension of this thought is that by training, interest and vocation the long term care administrator is the appropriate person to address ethical issues relative to management and leadership in long term care. In a nursing home, quality of life issues are addressed 24 hours a day and seven days a week. Ethical conduct during this long course of care is a most important set of actions; maybe even more important than those actions that are taken at terminus.

Therefore, ethical conduct or the absence of such conduct as it affects the well-being of a resident on a day-to-day basis has precedent over bioethical decisions made at the end phase of life. The intense focus of bioethics on issues concerning death or "right to life" has obscured ethical considerations of the caregivers during the life of the resident!

My contention is that ethics in administration must permeate the day to day activity of the administrator. More importantly, the daily decisions, big and small, must be construed in an ethical context. This cuts back to our efforts in this textbook to make administration patient-centered. If we follow this trend of thought, we must conclude that each and every decision we make, whether directly or indirectly related to patient well-being has an ethical connotation that must be adhered to.

How can each of these many and varied decisions be construed as being ethical in nature, we may ask. In order to respond to this question appropriately, we must firmly accept the basic premise that quality of life in a long-term care facility is equal to or more important than the quality of that which takes place at the time of death. If we accept this as a basic principle, then those decisions that contribute to the individual's day to day well-being must be as ethically grounded as those decisions that relate to life support systems, extension of life or the right to die. When we realize that even the smallest decision in some way affects the total psychosocial well-being of the people in our care, we must accept this as a truism. But because so many of our decisions are too remotely connected to a patient's well-being, we do not see the totality. It is very important to realize that the quality of life of a person being cared for is a composite of many components even though small routine decisions do not appear to affect this quality of life. They do become *part of the mosaic* that creates the quality of life. In many cases the whole is much greater than the sum of the individual parts in terms of the many decisions that an administrator may make.

Therefore, we are able to say that an administrative decision to allocate resources from a management viewpoint, is a decision that directly affects the total well-being of the person being cared for, and that viewed from a day to day quality of life standpoint, has every bit the ethical merit as a decision on life or death or life support.

Philosophical Ethicists

It is of interest at this point to delve into a somewhat academic, but not archean, component of ethics. This incursion will allow us to have broadly defined approaches that have historically been common in the field, but without particular definition or labeling.

Deontological Modes of Reasoning

This form of ethical thought maintains that there is more to ethics than just addressing the value of the end result. In other words, a great focus rests with the means by which end results are produced.

Business ethics, when academically defined, think it wrong to lie, cheat, steal, in other methodological activities regardless of the ultimate outcome. Therefore, because the methodology is wrong the action itself is wrong even though the consequences may be not considered bad. This form of thinking is surprisingly close to traditional religious ethical analysis, in the Protestant and Jewish faiths particularly, and in various secular liberal viewpoints expressed by early English philosophers, such as Locke and Hobbes.

Consequentialist Mode of Reason

Under this form of ethical thinking, common in the medical profession, actions are evaluated strictly on the basis of the consequences they produce. It is not to say that methodology and those acts that lead up to a consequence are totally out of the realm of evaluation, but there is a primacy in the thought process that, in its simplest form, states that the end is more important than the means.

The contrast here, then, would be in putting side by side what may be considered as contradictory philosophies of decision making and evaluation of ethical conduct. Insomuch as medical conduct may be viewed as different from business conduct in the health world, the contrasts of these two approaches may appear to be a conflict, and may in itself, need rationalizing for them to both coexist in a health/ethical milieu.

The Administrator as a Double Agent

One of the most important ethical conflicts to be brought to the surface is that of the double agent role created when a professional is hired by the corporation to serve the corporation's interest. The professional, be he administrator or other health professional, is through his training and professional standards, also an advocate for the patient or recipient of care. The conflict of these two roles inherent in the administrator's position, defines the double agent problem, which has many parallels throughout the health system, and is not exclusively a problem of the administrator of the service. Throughout this text we have been focusing on patient-oriented management decisions, yet we all recognize the prevalence of system or institution-oriented management decisions. Rationalizing that the success of ultimate patient care rests with the stability and successful functioning of the system, system-oriented decisions very often prevail. Most of the time it is difficult (except in very small organizations) to track administrative decisions to the patient level due to the complexity of the intervening organizational dynamics. Certainly an unstable, unsuccessful organization in the long run is deleterious to direct patient care, so that the primacy of the administrator as a corporate representative in this context has merit. In situations where the corporate representative has decisions that relate to profitability vis à vis other elements of organizational reward, the double agent concept becomes more onerous.

SOME QUESTIONS TO EXPLORE

Are ethical management decisions the same as moral management decisions?

How does the deontological and consequentialist modes of reasoning relate to management of a long term care service?

What is an ethical platitude and how does it relate to the ethics of management?

Could the professional ethics of the facility's staff differ from the ethical standards of the patients or their families?

What management decisions have clear ethical guidelines and which have unclear or ambiguous ones?

Community
and Governmental
Relationships

Administrators of long term care facilities have relationships with a variety of federal and state agencies. In this chapter we will begin to define specific areas where these governmental bodies interface with the average long term care facility so that the administrator has the opportunity to be prepared, and to make these contacts successful.

LOCAL GOVERNMENT

Every long term care facility must comply with all of the laws of the local jurisdiction. While by option or by mutual agreement local jurisdictions may defer to the state or federal government the endorsement of certain regulations, basic services such as sanitation, fire, police, street maintenance, zoning, and waste removal are very often subject to local control. By and large these issues are not of significance to the administrator in relation to his involvement with the state and federal regulatory bodies. Nevertheless, it behooves administration to be in compliance with all local ordinances. It may be advantageous to pursue the relationships on a local level as part of a community linkage program that more intimately relates the nursing home to the local community or, at least, the governmental part of that local community.

These relationships become very important when plans for expansion are discussed, or when there are major changes in local government services or service regulation such as garbage disposal, utilities or street maintenance. Local enforcement varies not just by geographic area, but also by degree of urbanization. A rule of thumb when dealing with issues that might be enforced at one or more levels of government, such as fire safety, is that the most restrictive regulatory guidelines must rule the day. It is very common to have a much stronger enforcement of certain service areas at the federal level than at the local level. Normally the state also has more stringent requirements than local government.

STATE REGULATORY RELATIONSHIPS

The most common interaction with the regulatory process is with the state regulatory agencies. The most significant of these bodies is the state hospital licensure, which is responsible for the enforcement of all regulations that are required by Medicaid and Medicare.

In order to insure that we cover the most significant interaction between government and administrator, let us divide these relationships into planning, licensure, service funding, and life safety.

HEALTH PLANNING

Health planning has been with us for many years and has been responsible for some of the better and worse system dynamics that has governed the direction of the long term care system. Title 15 of the Public Health Services Act which was aided by Public Law 93-641 required the establishment of Certificate of Need (C.O.N.) Program. The C.O.N. program which was administered by an approved state agency was primarily charged to govern the expansion of new institutional health services in the state. A cornerstone of the C.O.N. program was the rigid regulation of expansion of physical plant and acquisition of capital equipment. The program was created primarily for and directed to acute hospitals' capital investments. However, almost as an afterthought long term care was pulled in and governed to some degree by the same regulatory concepts that related to the acute hospital system. The C.O.N. program in most states rigidly controlled the expansion of both acute and long term facilities. It attempted to maintain bed patient ratios in certain geographic areas that fitted formulas usually agreed upon between the health and provider establishments. These formulas for hospital growth and development have been criticized for many years. Because of the political strength of individual hospitals or the hospital industry, even the tightly controlled C.O.N. program was unable to significantly stop the expansion of bed capacity in acute care. However, in long term it appeared to have been effective in deterring expansion and encouraging what is now a saturated system. I am using this term to describe the nursing home system which is currently running extremely high censuses throughout the country with the exception of certain select geographic areas. The construction of new facilities or expansion of older ones has been miniscule during these past five or six years and the high census throughout the field has been a decided disadvantage to the elderly person who is seeking, of necessity, admission to a nursing home. Because of this "no growth" phenomenon, the nursing homes have been able to exert greater political leverage on reimbursement regulation and service delivery than if they had to compete for patients because of the high vacancy factor. From the elderly person's standpoint, the high census has yielded fewer options and has created situations in most urban areas where the indigent elderly has the least array of choices when institutional services are needed. In many aras, the indigent population must go to the lower quality facilities, and, very often to a facility that is far away from their homes. These unfortunate circumstances are not all the fault of the C.O.N. programs, but, a reflection of a system mentality which believed that controlling the growth of nursing homes would advantage elderly persons by, among other things, forcing the development of non-institutional service systems. This has not happened to a significant degree. What has happened is that the population of elderly who bona fide-ly need skilled nursing has grown significantly while the institutional system has not. Thus creating a service gap that may widen further in the future.

The C.O.N. program is being phased out, but, the mentality that was responsible for stopping the growth of the industry in the face of increasing growth projections for the elderly population still exists. For all intents and purposes, tens of thousands of institutional beds will be needed by the end of this century. How planning agencies will allow this growth through the state's new regulations is a matter of conjecture. Some new laws are being created that will allow expansion by organizations to take place with few if any obstacles, and, will encourage the growth of the system by offering new economic incentives in the form of reimbursement, low-cost loans and/or new tax advantages to attract capital. This is similar to the circumstances in the early '60s that created the proprietary nursing home system in the first place. While there is every reason to believe that the institutional compo-nent of the long term system will expand substantially by the end of the cen-tury relatively unencumbered by governmental planning agencies; there is no assurance that this expansion will be equally balanced between pro-prietary, non-profit and public sector, nor that the quality of care will be any more improved with this larger institutional base.

State health planning agencies which implement federal planning regu-lations are also involved in the approval of a myriad of other elements to health service expansion. For example, most health planning departments rigidly control any changes that take place to the physical plant of a health facility, particularly if that change relates to a space occupied or involved with patient care. The involvement of state health planning with physical plant modifications in the long term care system varies from state to state. Their efforts to assure a safe and appropriate environment are noteworthy and have contributed greatly to improved institutional environments by providing for better safety, appropriate space and acceptable construction standards. The Office of State Health Planning is usually charged with the responsibility for the enforcement of the Occupational Safety & Health Act as well as state and federal fire standards. The future of health planning will no doubt retain an emphasis on physical plant and capital equipment. Yet, there is some indication that health delivery systems, or in the case of long term care local integrated service systems will become a *major focus* of state planning efforts instead of being tangentially related to the emphasis on capital issues.

LICENSURE AND CERTIFICATION

As we discussed, in the history of long term care, the refinement of the licensure and certification process is a distillation of those similar activities in acute care. At this point it is truly impossible to operate a skilled nursing facility without being licensed. Although licensure requirements vary from state to state, the requirement that facilities receiving funding from Title 18 or 19 be in compliance with federal regulations mandates a significant degree of uniformity throughout the country. While there are still facilities which do not receive funding through these governmental programs, they still must be in compliance with the state licensure laws, which in most cases have been brought up to parity with Federal regulations. So at present, there is little advantage, if any, in not complying with Federal standards.

In some cases certification, a process handled separately from licensing, may be more difficult to acquire than licensure. It is possible for a facility to meet the conditions of licensure but not be certifiable to receive payment under the Medicaid or Medicare program.

Usually the Federal government will contract with the State to inspect facilities for Medicare regulation compliance. The Feds periodically audit the State's work in this regard and occasionally will perform the survey themselves. Another "inspection" may take place to determine whether or not the residents in a skilled nursing facility or intermediate care facility are at the right acuity level for that facility. Some call this a *level of care determination*. It is usually made through either a state office or federal office by nurses who review utilization patterns and acuity profiles of the residents. This separate study is often linked with the licensing and certification because of its analysis of certain care components that are also part of licensing regulations.

SAFETY AND DISASTER PREPAREDNESS

Under the Occupational Safety and Health Act of 1970 (OSHA), it is required that each employer furnish to his employees a hazard-free environment which complies with standards set forth under this act. Compliance further requires substantial amounts of documentation. Although these are federal programs, the administration and enforcement of these standards is usually through a state agency. While there may be separate OSHA inspectors, the state departments of fire safety promulgate the criteria of the life-safety code, which was prepared by the National Fire Protection Association. The enforcement of fire safety can and is often done by local and state regulatory agencies. Under normal circumstances, state standards take precedence over local standards. Both state and local agencies attempt to survey the facility for compliance at least yearly.

ECONOMIC INTERACTIONS

The primary source of funding of long term care is the Medicaid Title 19 program. Approximately $50 billion a year flow from the government into skilled nursing facilities. Approximately 46% of all nursing home income comes from this program and approximately 3% of nursing home income comes from Title 18 Medicare program. The remainder flows from private pay sources, a small percentage of which is manifested in various forms of third party private insurance programs.

The primary contact between the government in this case is through fiscal intermediaries which will be discussed in another chapter. The billing mechanisms of Title 18 and 19 reimbursement plans are complex, and any administrator soon finds out that the "life blood" of any organization depends on his ability to assure the smooth and timeliness, if now flawless, submission of billings. Many have found out that the least inattention to the details of these complex funding programs will cost the administrator, not only sorely needed income, but possibly his job.

REGULATORY RELATIONSHIPS

Not all the relationships that confront an administrator of a long term care facility are regulatory. Many are with community resources that offer great opportunity for economic as well as political support. The administrator who understands a community's fabric and is able to maximize the resources within that community will be able to enhance the rendering of that facility's quality of care. Most certainly, the use of these community resources will allow him to supply benefits to his residents that normal operating revenue sources could not provide.

The most often overlooked resources are those that are closest to the nursing facility; for example neighborhood associations and nearby churches, community centers, and schools. To expand this thought a little further, most communities have a chamber of commerce, community action councils, and local housing authorities. The knowledge of youth groups and how to reach them and of the variety of service organizations, such as Lions and Rotary, is vital to the successful long term operation of a nursing facility.

In other words, to function successfully the skilled nursing facility must be part of the fabric of its community. The development of positive relationships with these varied groups implies something quite germane to the success of the operation of a nursing home. It suggests that the nursing home should be without walls or barriers. It is not only a great opportunity for communication, but of access and involvement with these groups. While difficult to accept, this invitation to the community and its successful implementation may be the single most important factor that will support the organization through good times and bad.

The open facility described may seem logical, but, in fact, has been resisted by private sector organizations for some time. This putting off of the community has created a schism between the institution and the community and in many cases has developed an adversarial relationship. If one were to view this negative relationship to its full extent, one would see that it encourages a combative attitude by advocacy groups and creates artificial barriers to community involvement with your program. It also fuels the fire of the facility's negative image within the community at large.

More importantly, it deprives the resident of the nursing facility of the human contact with community members who would render service to the facility. In our discussion of the psychosocial model, we found that bringing the community into the nursing home (a form of mainstreaming) had a significant impact on the quality of life. By the same token, the rejection of community resources and a construction of an artificial barrier to keep "them" out puts the administrator at a decided disadvantage in his efforts to administer an already-problematic institution.

While the responsibility to develop these specific relationships may fall on the shoulders of different people within the nursing home's organization, the administrator is ultimately accountable for the success or failure of this aspect of his duty. Once the administrator understands this unique responsibility, it must then be assigned to other key staff members. In order to be effective the training and education of nursing home staff in this community linkage process takes a great deal of finesse, some time and some resources. But the payoff is tremendous. Each staff member has the potential to be a goodwill ambassador to some component of the community. Whether it's the administrator with direct contact to the chamber of commerce, or an aide's relationship with her neighborhood church, the collective impact on the nursing home is great. This utilization of community resources, which takes on the shape of a volunteer program, will be discussed further under internal management.

Survey and Compliance

At the core of the administrative function lies the administrator's ability to comply with state, federal and local regulations. At this point the regulatory surveillance of long term care, particularly nursing homes, is more intense than with any other aspect of the health and human service system. While the chapter will focus on survey and compliance as it relates to skilled nursing facilities it is important to realize that the general principles we will discuss are applicable to all other services in long term care. As the other components of the continuum grow in size and importance, there no doubt will be increased effort at regulatory control and a concomitant need for administrators to thoroughly understand all aspects of regulatory implementation and compliance.

As we discussed in the previous chapter, there is often great inconsistency between the needs and demands of consumer groups and the regulations that are actually implemented in a facility and enforced by the regulatory agencies. Nevertheless, each state has some agency that is responsible for licensing and certification. The purpose of this responsibility is to ensure quality health services to each resident throughout their system. These regulations must be enforced regardless of the patient's economic status, race, age or sex. While there are wide statutory variations in the nature of survey and compliance, we will define certain common characteristics that, if not ideal, are at least a standard throughout the country.

Beyond the basic regulatory goal of the inspection agency is its task of producing consistent, accurate and useful evaluations of each facility. These evaluations are used to determine if the facility will qualify for the Medicare and Medicaid programs. The state must first certify a facility in order for it to be qualified to accept residents covered by these programs. Thus, the process of licensing and certification will be affected by the professional makeup and operating philosophies of the surveying bodies. The state will make an effort to hire and train people for its survey teams who have academic backgrounds and work experience in the health field. The ultimate goal would be that nurses will survey nursing departments, administrators will survey administration, and paramedics will survey for their particular paramedical specialty.

It is possible to view the role of the inspection teams as a consultative one; that is, to direct the state surveyors toward the advisement of the facility's management. If, on the other hand, the state's operating policy stresses the enforcement component of survey and compliance, the relationship to management will be quite clearly adversarial.

It is clear that there is room for both of these functions in the survey, although to pursue either of these possibilities to the extreme would compromise the effect of the entire process.

Historically, the consultative approach has been the most commonly used. But institutional abuse of the regulations and findings of negligent resident care mandated a more assertive enforcement approach. To combine the two roles—advisement and enforcement—should be the optimal goal of the survey agency. Unfortunately, the determination of which role should be emphasized is often a political one, or in some cases a product of public and media intervention.

STRUCTURE OF SURVEY

Each skilled nursing facility is visited periodically by a team of specially trained surveyors who determine the extent to which the facility has complied with the state and federal regulations governing their operation. The survey team will hopefully record its notes in accordance with the same resident-centered bias that management should be pursuing. While these surveys are conducted in an assertive adversarial manner, it is decidedly to the advantage of the administrator to have formal but positive relationships with the survey team. This attitude of formal, positive and congenial support should exist at all levels of nursing home operation. It is not unheard-of to have "serious" deficiencies noted by the surveyors for no other reason than that an open conflict has erupted between the survey team and the hospital staff.

Agencies responsible for conducting these surveys are very often underfunded. Surveyors are not paid at a level equal to their significant responsibility and expertise. Also there is often some question about their training, which varies, and in some states is less than adequate. Given these factors it is easier to understand the subjective nature of the interpretation of regulations as they relate to any specific facility. Since at the very core of the process of surveillance is the suspected existence of a violation, there is normally little or no component of the survey that offers a positive expression for commendatory performance.

The heart of the survey centers around the facility's policies and procedures. Therefore, it is vital that these policies and procedures be designed around regulatory requirements. The pivotal function of the survey is the compliance with the facility's own policies and procedures. There is also an emphasis on how policies and procedures are formulated and subsequently modified or updated according to regulatory requirements. Should it not be possible to comply with a particular regulation, there is usually a waiver clause or program flexibility clause that allows approval of this omission by the state. It is to the administrator's decided advantage to periodically review and reconcile regulations with operating policies and procedures; and make sure that the staff concerned with these policies and procedures are educated in their implementation on a periodic basis throughout the year. Unfortunately because of the variety of day-to-day crises that utilize the time and energy of staff and management, policies are often shelved and referred to only at time of inspections. The ability of an administrator to utilize policies and procedures (as they relate to regulations) on an active basis often determines his or her ability to do well on the surveys.

The state has a variety of enforcement tools at its disposal. Fines can be levied, and licensure can be threatened, by either suspension or revocation. If the facility is totally negligent on many levels, there are ways to place it in receivership to protect the resident. Another enforcement tool, often used, is to remove the facility's certification to participate in the Medicare and Medicaid programs.

The goal of the enforcement is to produce, initially, the immediate correction of stated violations or to subsequently establish the facility's willingness to permanently prevent any re-occurrence.

Once again—throughout the survey process, total cooperation with the inspecting body should be the rule. At the end of the survey it is advisable to have a verbal review of the survey team's findings prior to the written report. This will allow the facility the opportunity to present information that may have been overlooked and will allow the state to explain its rationale in some detail. The next step is the written survey listing in detail the specific regulatory code that was violated. The facility must now write what is called a plan of correction. This plan of correction is best made on the same form where the written citations are noted. The plan of correction should include specifically what action will be taken to reverse the violation, and an anticipated timeline for implementation. The state then has the option of accepting or not accepting the plan of correction. If they do not accept the plan, it is their responsibility to so inform the facility, and set their own limits on the period in which corrective actions must be taken. It should be assumed that the state inspection team will return at an appropriate time to determine if these actions have taken place. If for some reason a corrective action on a particular violation is *not* possible, there must be a waiver or a special state acknowledgement of this unique situation.

ADMINISTRATIVE HEARING

Should there be a violation that directly affects the health safety or security of a resident, there may be need for a higher level of adjudication. In some states there are fine systems for this type of problem; however, it is important that the administrator seek to deal directly with the licensing body at an administrative level higher than that of the surveyor. This may or may not be a legal hearing, but it will be a planned hearing where the ramifications of the violation can be explored in greater depth. It is hoped that a resolution of the problem as it relates to either the regulation or the plan of correction will be dealt with at the highest possible level of administrative authority.

Should it appear that an administrative hearing will not solve the problem, the matter may require a more sophisticated approach. In these situations it may be advisable to seek appropriate legal counsel for advice.

QUALITY OF CARE

The relationship between survey process and quality of care is a subject of a great deal of debate. Astute officials are the first to admit that this form of survey is primarily designed to protect people from a variety of negative possibilities rather than create positive realities. From their viewpoint this punitive or adversarial viewpoint is the successful approach to dealing with potential care violations.

But what of quality of life? How does the "paper compliance" with the regulations relate to the day-to-day living quality of the resident? Is the state confusing quality of care with quality of life? There are many examples of facilities which present flawless patterns to the inspection team, yet whose sterile environment and rigid medical structure still lend themselves at best, to a mediocre quality of life.

What we see then is an unfortunate conflict between the psychosocial model and the medical model. If our analysis is correct, the medical model is used as the springboard for the regulatory process. Therefore, it is quite possible to have a facility that is in total compliance yet lacking in any of those essentials deemed necessary for an enhanced quality of life. This lack of consideration for the psychosocial need contributes to the public image of a nursing home being a place to store bodies, and makes efforts to truly improve the quality of life there, frustrating for those upon whom this responsibility falls.

During the '80s, regulation will move from "paper compliance" to some form of "outcome" measurement. While the intent of this shift is admirable, preliminary evaluations of this new system using "patient assessment" indicates reliance on the medical model and a continuation of a flawed regulatory process.

For the administrator who understands the limitations of the regulatory process and wishes to strive for those levels of quality not mandated by this system, there are many opportunities to do so. The ability to improve a facility by bringing to it vitality, warmth and humanity must start from the leadership (or the administration) of the facility and must permeate the recruitment and selection process of individuals hired to work there. The philosophy of offering improved quality of life to the residents of a nursing facility must truly permeate the entire organization.

Throughout the country there are many examples of successful institutional living. There is much evidence that an elderly person or her family will opt for institutional living over the loneliness and isolation that some elderly lifestyles create. Regardless of the mechanistic determination of the regulatory process, when a person is settled in a nursing facility that space becomes the elderly person's home, or his biosphere, and is every bit as important and valuable to him as anything else he has had in the past. This territorial precept of the elderly nursing home resident should take primacy in the administrator's thinking; that regardless of the economic or system limitations necessary to comply with regulations, the space occupied by that elderly resident must be sacrosanct, and appropriate services and supports must be offered to allow that person to enjoy life to the limits of her capabilities.

During the past decade, significant improvement has been made in the nursing home system. Most of this improvement has been related to the training, upgrading and licensure of administrators and to the upgrading of the nurse assistants and other workers by requiring certifications or other forms of upgrading programs.

In other words, regulatory compliance is just a starting point. It's the beginning of the arduous process the administrator accepts as his responsibility for developing a truly positive environment where growth and independence are possible, where self-esteem and dignity are maintained, and where hope in the future is present.

Fiscal Intermediaries

When the creation of massive governmental funding programs for health care began, the difficulty in the mechanical transfer of governmental funds to the provider became a problem. The decision to administer the finances of these major programs, without further expanding federal and state bureaucracies, led to the information of non-governmental fiscal managing entities known as fiscal intermediaries. The most common of these organizations nationwide are Blue Cross, Blue Shield, Mutual of Omaha, and other large well known organizations that had a history of involvement in the health insurance arena.

In fulfilling the complex responsibility of transmitting government funds to providers of service, these private sector organizations essentially convert state and federal law into organizational operating policies and procedures.

The importance of the administrator's role in dealing with fiscal intermediaries and understanding their function must be emphasized. The billing system for the Medicare and Medicaid programs is one of the most complex ever devised; and it is made that much more difficult because of the relatively unsophisticated business machinery existing in many nursing homes. Above and beyond the labyrinth bookkeeping required, it should be understood that the policies and procedures of the fiscal intermediary, viewed from the standpoint of the LTC administrator, are tantamount to law, and serve as inflexible operating guidelines for the receipt of money.

TRUE INTERMEDIARY OR AGENT

The major misconception of the role of the fiscal intermediary is that they are a true intermediary between provider and state. Some think that their role "in the middle" is that of an ombudsman who adjudicates the differences that may arise between provider and state, and then makes payment to the provider based on that adjudicated decision. While the standards promulgated by the fiscal intermediary are not replications of state and federal standards, the fiscal intermediary is a contractual agent of the state and has a vested interest in representing the state's viewpoint. From the administrator's standpoint, it should be realized that there is an ongoing polemic in process between provider of service and payer of government funds. There is no reason to believe that there should be total agreement since the goals of these two bodies are simply not the same.

To sum up: The state must comply with the regulations that have been derived from the law, and must also protect the utilization of public funds. The fiscal intermediary which contracts for the administration and transmittal of these funds must take that same viewpoint. Therefore, in reality, the administrator is dealing with an agent of the state that has as its mandate a most conservative and restrictive interpretation of federal law and regulation.

If we accept this mandate as a responsibility of a contract agent of the state, then we must also include the possibility that the fiscal intermediary may interpret state regulations in an even more restrictive posture than the original intention. It should be noted, in this context, that even though the fiscal intermediaries translate the same federal and state regulations, they may have different organizational policies and procedures that may appear to run contrary to the basic rationale of the original federal law. The interpretations may even differ between intermediaries.

What this means is that the policies, procedures and standards of the fiscal intermediary are not immutable; quite to the contrary. They are subject to challenge at a variety of different levels. The history of the development of the long term care system from the standpoint of reimbursement is rife with examples of nonpayment of claims by the fiscal intermediary. While there are many reasons for these nonpayments, the responsibility is usually placed on the provider. Some states anticipate these rejections to the extent that these claim rejections are factored into their own operating budgets. Therefore, it would appear to be disadvantageous to the state, which has already incorporated rejected claims into its budget, to devise ways of making the payment system more advantageous to the provider, since it is the provider who is usually forced to absorb the loss.

SYSTEM SUMMARY

In essence, the provider of service, (the nursing home in this case) delivers the service to a resident and bills the state through the fiscal intermediary. The billing process includes a complex series of forms overlaid with various tightly structured time constraints. However, when a bill is submitted to the fiscal intermediary, there is no legally-required response time for the intermediary's payment of these bills. It is quite possible, even after efficiently handling the billing procedure, to wait weeks or months for the repayment. This delay in cash flow must be factored into the problems of fiscal management since the absence of this operating income could cripple the ability to maintain a consistent and stable service delivery within the facility. Claim payment delays and rejections of billings (later overturned in court) have been the cause of many long term care facility failures, and constitute a deterrent for development of new nursing homes by small partnerships or sole proprietors.

In the planning of a long term care facility, claim rejection and delays in payments must be factored into both the opening phase of the organization and, then continually, into the operational phase. This operational "float" is a crucial factor in determining the economic health of an organization.

Many operations have been crippled because this has not been taken properly into account.

THE CHALLENGE

A major area of conflict develops when bills are rejected or claims for specific services are denied. Intrinsic to the relationship between the provider and the fiscal intermediary is a system of appeals that allows the provider to challenge the denial. It is important to know that, depending on the value of the claim being denied, the provider may extend his appeal to the courts. What is very often found is that because the internal policies and procedures developed by the fiscal intermediary are different enough from the basic intent of the law and governmental regulation that there is a good opportunity to resolve the issue legally in favor of the provider. The fiscal intermediary may exaggerate the standards of the government and, in that case, penalize the provider of service (in this case the nursing home). It is very important that the administrator understand this aspect of his facility's relationship with the fiscal intermediary. Adverse action on part of the fiscal intermediary could easily disqualify attempts to offer quality of care to the residents of the nursing home. Therefore the administrator must scrutinize his billing procedures very closely. Since operating income is the lifeblood of the SNF, these procedures must work flawlessly. Otherwise, they inevitably will lead to the loss or delay of needed operating revenues, as well as the expenditure of considerable amounts of administrative time and energy.

Planning and Development

OVERVIEW

Since the terms planning and development are used or abused in many ways, we may as well recognize that we are talking about two distinctly different processes. Therefore, for the sake of this text, we will define these terms and develop the rest of this chapter based on those particular definitions. We must recognize, also, that in the past decade since planning has come of age, there are many permutations to the planning process that may, at first blush, appear to contradict each other.

Planning as a discipline in the health field began to develop a formalized structure in the mid-'60s when most urban areas in the country created some form of planning authority that was usually designed as a consultative body. The primary thrust of health planning was the recognition, even in the mid-'60s, of the enormous misuse of resources that existed in the health field. The primary incentive for formalized health planning arose out of the misallocation of resources that existed in the acute hospital system.

The first and most specific concerns about the misallocation of these resources related to the purchase and replication within any particular community of very expensive capital equipment (cobalt therapy units in hospitals just a few blocks apart) and the virtually uncontrolled expansion of hospital physical plants. The evils of these reported misallocations of resources were that the enormous deficits incurred by hospitals had to be made up by either the support community of the hospital or by third party payers, who were noting a radical increase in hospital costs during this period.

This precipitous rise in acute hospital costs has been attributed to a variety of things; such as, excessive capital expenditures, exorbitant management costs, high salaries or incomes for physicians, significant increase in the salaries of hospital workers, etc. Towards the end of the '60s, health planning formalized around the effort to control the acute hospital system.

In the early '70s health planning throughout the country became a part in the approval cycle of all hospitals and health facilities. It was no longer advisory or consultative, but now had a decision making role in the control of the expansion of the hospital system. In most jurisdictions the approval of this agency was needed before a hospital could expand, buy major pieces of equipment, or do a large remodeling project.

Towards the end of the '70s federal law created the Health System Agencies throughout the country, which defined health planning in a structurally new way, purportedly giving the major decision making authority to local communities. The boards of these HSAs were composed of providers and consumers, the consumers in control, and the concept of certificate of need (CON) was developed as the vehicle to control the expansion of hospitals. For a variety of reasons, primarily funding issues and questionable success after five years of operation, the HSA system by and large disappeared from the scene and the strength of the CON changed also primarily to local or state option. In essence, health planning in terms of its effect on the hospital systems expansion, is not too far from where it was in the mid-'60s; it's come a full circle.

While any planner who may read the previous two paragraphs is probably grimacing at the somewhat simplistic, abbreviated history of health planning, I think it's important that we even go into health planning from a conceptual standpoint that may put planning and operations in a more palatable context.

In most fields there is a schism between its academic and practitioner's sides. There is always a conflict between basic scientists and the teachers of that science; between academic engineers and people working as engineers in industry. In the field of health, there is no less a gap. The field of planning is viewed by practitioners as being populated by people who have little or no experience in the field. Their ideas are abstract and impractical and are often doomed to failure from the writing of the first word. Point of fact, planners are often trained in college and go directly after graduate levels of training into important planning roles without ever having experienced the realities of the field. The practitioner views the planner as one who deals in improbabilities, and who is never around to reap the benefits or the failures of his plan. Practitioners in the health field who have been responsible for implementation of plans feel that the failures in the evolution of the health field have been due to faulty planning and are somewhat aggrieved at the planning profession as a whole. They feel that the planner should be made to be part of the implementation team for any plan and should be responsible for its success or failure.

The planner, on the other hand, views the practitioner as the primary cause of the ills of the system. He feels that field experience isn't that important because it has been translated in academic fashion into the coursework material used in his training. He thoroughly believes that the failure of any of his plans is due to the poor implementation capability of the practitioner, and is the first one to seek an upgrading of the practitioner's standards and capabilities.

To the degree that this attitude is pervasive in the health field, both sides to this question have made entreaties to the other side to attempt to bridge the gap. Planners have gone into the field for internships and special training. Practitioners have taken courses in planning and have sat on planning bodies. After two decades of evolution, planners and practitioners may be closer now than ever before. Nevertheless the old biases still exist and it should be the responsibility of all parties concerned to bridge these gaps and utilize the combined wisdom and knowledge of planner and practitioner alike.

LONG TERM CARE

Long term care, more specifically skilled nursing care, became involved tangentially as a tag-end to health planning in the late 1960s. Regulating the nursing home system was really an afterthought, and something considered much less important than planning's primary focus—the acute hospital. Because planning for the nursing home system had such a low level of importance, it was not initially perceived that the planning theory applied to acute hospitals was totally inappropriate for the skilled nursing system. Acute and skilled nursing are part of two greatly different systems as I have explained before, and to develop a set of planning standards that were applicable to skilled nursing required a great understanding of the dynamics of the skilled nursing system.

Unfortunately the knowledge of the dynamics of the skilled nursing system was not known to the planners, and those structures created by health planning that related to nursing homes were essentially replications of guidelines utilized for acute hospitals.

The incorporation of the long term care system (primarily the nursing home system) in the same technology that governed the planning modalities for acute care was faulty in many respects. The most important differences between the system was the market dynamics caused by the paradoxical confrontation between the nonprofit system, (i.e., the hospitals) and the proprietary system (i.e., the skilled nursing homes). We also have to recognize that there are a significant number of nonprofit nursing homes and a growing number of proprietary acute hospitals. Nevertheless, the market dynamics in terms of supply and demand is governed by these two quite different market systems.

Another major difference between the systems that caused a great deal of conflict in health planning was that while the acute hospital system may have been guilty of misallocation of resources and rampant cost increase, the skilled nursing system was, by and large, a controlled system. The primary source of revenues for the patients in the skilled nursing system was Medicaid, which, by and large, was a flat rate per diem system that rose incrementally very slowly in an historical relationship with the acute hospitals, which had a cost related reimbursement system. In any event, health planning for skilled nursing homes incorporated in its basic dogma certain very high census standards (in some states as high as 95%) before expansion would be allowed in any designated area.

A certificate of need, therefore, would be granted only if the census would be 95% or greater. The development of that system would be contained substantially. In point of fact, the planning process that was originally started to prevent inappropriate use of resources was not juxtaposed in the marketplace and created a very unhealthy environment for the elderly person.

The reason was, that the high levels of census required before expansion could occur generated a "saturated" system. By saturated system I mean one that, in this case, had a very low vacancy, so that in any particular area an elderly person who needed to have a nursing bed would find that most of the good facilities were full, and that the only beds that were available were in a lesser, lower quality facility. Because the system was saturated with a high census, nursing homes no longer felt the need to be competitive by offering higher quality, more varied services. In essence, they controlled the market. This control allowed the nursing home system to cream off the private pay patient and triage, or exclude, the indigent patient or the heavy care patient. This adverse selection process caused the indigent or Medicaid elderly patient to have a marked disadvantage in that the only beds available were only in the more inferior facilities.

Not only would the indigent patient find that he or she could not get into the better facilities, in many urban areas because of the saturated condition, they were forced into going to the outlying areas just to get a bed, thus separating them from their families and social networks. The tragedy of the saturated nursing home system, which sent these elderly people very often into other counties, was augmented by the rapid inflation in construction costs that took place in the latter '70s, which made it economically very costly for new nursing homes to be built. As we pointed out earlier, the actual bed stock of the nursing home industry stabilized, and has only shown minute growth since the late '70s. The disadvantage to the elderly was never a concern to planners. Now the market was controlled by the dominant proprietary interests that have, to a great extent, amalgamated into large corporate entities. In the mid-'80s, therefore, an unbalanced system exists, which unfortunately has been a great disservice to our elderly.

What we have described is an overview of planning which will serve as a foundation for the planning and development which takes place within any component of the long term care system. When one seeks to address the internal needs for planning, one must find a logical interface with the external planning environment.

INTERNAL PLANNING

At one time, in the not too distant past, a great deal was made out of long term planning. Long term was viewed usually three to five years and in some instances by more stable and self-assured organizations, as long as ten years in advance.

Intermediate plans were usually thought of as one to three years and short range would be for a fiscal year. Then at some point, strategic planning came into the jargon and its next of kin, a tactical plan. Right now, strategic planning appears to be the jargon in control of planners' mentality, and because system dynamics are changing so radically, long term care plans rarely exceed five years. The term "development" is usually defined as the process that takes place after planning is completed, one that implements the plan up to the day the service is open and operative.

While it is very often the responsibility of the administrator to develop a plan, there is an equal chance that outside consultants will be brought in to handle the project, or that a committee of the board will become the planning committee with administrator as the lead professional. This initial structuring of the planning leadership is crucial to the ultimate success of the plan.

PLANNING INCENTIVES

With this very brief overview of the external planning environment and several comments on the basic organization, let us look more closely at those motives that are the stimulus for the planning process. First of all, we have to assume that a plan initiated by a governmental agent, say for example, the Office of State Health Planning, or a regional or local planning agency, begin that plan because it is their legal mandate and their raison d'être. So planning, as a basic function of an agency, in itself appears to be a motive. In reality, however, as history has demonstrated, it is usually a response to a variety of other factors, and is not usually initiated in a vacuum. This view is even more appropriate in the case of long term care, which is rarely a focus of official planning agencies. Long term care has only recently been on the horizon and is a very fragile entity. Planners who are trained in public health or planning an acute hospital system, have not demonstrated in the past any significant knowledge or expertise in long term care or of specific factors which would indicate that a needs analysis in any particular geographic area should take place. Certainly, senior housing may be an exception and there are sporadic examples throughout the country of focus studies for the need for a particular service.

By and large, long term care planning from the standpoint of official agencies who are designated to develop systems, has been sorely lacking. But let's go on a little further, to the front lines, and find out the motivation that would encourage private proprietary or private nonprofit to develop a plan for their organization.

PROFITABILITY

I have already mentioned that a most significant difference between the acute system and the long term care system is the reality that long term care is primarily a proprietary system. Therefore, we must conclude that the most significant motivating force for planning long term care will be the profitability factor.

In the early '60s, it became quite evident that Medicare and Medicaid would be implemented. One of the most significant events that took place during this period was the incorporation, in the basic Medicare and Medicaid formula, of significant financial incentives to attract private capital. Public policy at that time was not directed at creating a mammoth, governmental, long term care system because public sector facilities caring for the aged and disabled had terrible reputations. Money was cheap and the construction industry was sophisticated. It was easy to envision a system that reduced the stress on the existing acute hospital and allowed for the institutional care of the elderly in the proprietary sector. The financial inducements were not only operational profitability, but significant returns on capital investment.

This incentive brought out sole proprietors, contractors, groups of physicians, small investment groups, and owners of board and care facilities who saw the opportunity to make a goodly profit. Planning consisted of doing a financial feasibility study of a nursing home with a projected census that incorporated existing reimbursement levels. These somewhat primitive studies seldom had any sound demographic data to support them. Initiated in a period when money was cheap and abundant, these feasibility studies were not scrutinized in any great depth by the lenders. Very often uncollateralized loans were made, and the only issue of concern was finding a site in an area reasonably close to an acute hospital. Planning, therefore, in the proprietary sense, was, and still is, directed towards the end of a traditional planning cycle, that is, the developmental phase.

Once the land had been secured, and the loans approved, the construction and the design could proceed with great haste. The plan, therefore, proceeded from an economic feasibility to development and implementation of services as soon as possible. There was rarely any attention paid to marketing because PR appeared to suffice at getting patients and referrals. Since the primary source of public relations was directed at physicians, very little information about the facility ever reached the public. If any one facility, once operating, showed significant profitability, a plan was initiated to build and operate another similar facility. What passed for the extension of the planning process was essentially no more than a replication of the initial effort in new locations.

Because of the proprietary sector's relatively easy access to money, broader views of planning were rarely necessary; the goal was to become operative as soon as possible, go directly to the source of patient referral, and promote the facility to that referral source. Towards the mid-'70s when the corporate chains began to expand in size, planning took on a new dimension, which was more closely allied with other industrial enterprises. Still the fulcrum of these planning efforts was the profitability of any enterprise and the utilization of existing cash flow and equity build-up to expand the corporation. Corporate planning at this level follows a traditional economic model of expansion that includes: economic feasibility of construction or acquisition; a quick shifting of resources to the site of profitability; a very concerted effort to get the variety of approvals needed to build a facility; standardized building plans; short construction periods; and movement into the competitive marketplace in that area, in the shortest possible time.

In the '80s, corporate skills at developing a marketing plan improved considerably. There was now available better base data about the demographics of any particular area, reasonably long track records for given facilities, and stabilized patterns of discharge and referral. Additionally, the technology of marketing nursing home services became more sophisticated and more acceptable to the public at large. Discharge sources were no longer the only source of referral, nor were physicians the primary target of advertising and public relations. Community networks became important even to proprietary entities and it became the responsibility of the administrator to understand and develop these community networks, so that referral of patients could come from a variety of directions (thus stabilizing the census of any given facility).

Regardless of the refinements in this development process that have emerged in the nursing home field over the past 20 years, the sole criteria for the beginning of a plan, whether it was acquisition of an existing facility, construction of a new one, or expansion had to do with its potential profitability.

DEMAND FOR SERVICE AS A MOTIVATOR

The second most important motivating factor in planning was the demand for the service. Obviously demand is an integral component of financial profitability, but we are looking at demand in a different way at this point. Many organizations will initiate a planning program strictly because of the demand for that particular service. In the long term care continuum the demand for different services may vary considerably in any community. It is, as we discussed in the previous chapter, one of the most difficult components to calculate in designing a continuum. The most obvious response to the demand has been in the nonprofit housing sector, where senior housing has been primarily initiated because of a real or perceived demand for service. The demand alone, regardless of economic considerations, will in these cases initiate a planning process. For most of the nonprofit sector involved in homes for the aging, demand also serves as the primary mover. In these cases, it is a very tightly-focused demand directed towards constituent populations that creates these organizations, whether they be religious, ethnic or fraternal.

In the case of nonprofit homes, the planning process continues for a longer time period because usually the group has a greater need to understand the long term demographics of its own small population. The most common examples of what used to be called long term planning, was found in nonprofit organizations when they were preparing to care for a specific population over the next 3, 5 or 10 years. The nonprofit sector can thus be justifiably used as a model of planning processes that (unlike the proprietary sector) extend beyond pure development.

NONPROFIT PLANNING MODELS

Using the nonprofit system as one which offers some examples of more complex planning programs, we should now at least recognize semantic differences in the description of planning. At one point in the recent past the idea of master planning was in vogue. This connoted long range planning, which by definition could be three years, five years or ten years or more. We have to recognize that up through the early 1970s, long range planning could be done for such lengthy periods of time because system change was very slow, and these changes themselves have proven to be one of the most important factors in validating any particular plan. Therefore, if a master plan was created in the '50s or '60s that conceived of a system dynamic that lasted 5 to 10 years, they were probably right on target. Systems changed much more slowly, making long term predictions much more reliable. Shifting to the '80s, the system dynamics has become very, very short-cycled; therefore long term masterplans become blue sky conjectures that lack reliability and validity. Since the mid-'70s, the health systems go through 3 to 5 year cycles of change that must be factored into the reality of a long term masterplan.

Somewhere along the line long term planning, or masterplanning, has become strategic planning, with much shorter timelines. From the standpoint of our discussion, let us call *strategic planning* both comprehensive and long range 3 to 5 years; let us call planning projects that need one to three years *mid-range planning*, and call shorter term planning (within one year) as *tactical planning*, dealing with those directly operational issues needed to implement components of midrange and strategic planning. Be sure, when entering a planning process, that all parties to the planning process are defining their terms in an agreed upon manner.

Certain basic guidelines can be used to set the parameters for mid range or strategic planning. Possibly the easiest are brick and mortar projects, which have reasonably predictable time-lines; that is, you can estimate the length of time between the basic organizational steps and groundbreaking, and with reasonable accuracy project the timeline between groundbreaking and opening day.

DEFINITION OF DEMAND

We've used the demographic projections of a specific constituent group as one example of demonstrating demand for institutional services. This is a traditional, but dangerously simplistic definition of demand that must be explored further.

Demand means different things to different people, and we must ask ourselves who is the demand being made upon? Is it a sponsoring organization that exists? Is it a community? Is it an amorphous and intangible demand? Is it a service-specific demand? Is demand defined by a certain specific number of people needing a clearly defined service? Is demand defined by waiting lists in existing facilities, by governmental statistics, by population trend projections?

It is very important to clarify the demand issue if you're going to respond to it in a planning mode. Recognizing that demand has many dimensions is an important beginning point. An analysis of demand and its different perspectives will assist you in more accurately planning both physical plant and program. It will also more clearly indicate who is responsible for meeting the demand. This first critical decision establishes the design for the entire planning process. The most common responsible party is the existing charitable organization that serves a specifically defined community. If this tight focus is not possible, there will be the necessity of pulling together community leaders, citizens, and interested parties of good faith. In other words, there has to be an initiating body to a planning project; either an existing body or one that has been newly created.

INTERNAL PLANNING

Now let me outline a planning process that we will develop in the rest of this chapter, recognizing that the initiating factor and the responsible party are of prime concern before this planning process can begin.

1. Identity phase
2. Market analysis phase
3. Project model phase
4. Fiscal analyses phase
5. Procedural processing phase
6. Design development phase
7. Construction phase
8. Implementation phase
9. Monitoring phase
10. Evaluation and change

IDENTITY PHASE

In my opinion, the identity phase is the most important part of the internal planning process. It is during this period that the planning body finds out who they are, what they're doing, who they are responsible to, and what their level of authority is. Most planning processes I have been involved with have had to go through a tortuous period of self-discovery, where individuals on a planning body define their own personal role and the group collectively becomes, through dialogue and analyses, an organizational structure. It is during this phase that it must decide its level of authority in everything from financial commitment to the involvement of any larger body they may represent. They must find out if they are an advisory group or a group that is empowered to carry the plan through to completion. They must decide whether they, as individuals, are buying into the product of the group or whether they represent vested interests that comprise different factions within a larger body. They must determine what approvals are needed beyond their level of decision making and who will make these approvals.

Concomitant with this "identity crisis" is the need to develop a mission statement that is, by consensus, acceptable to the group and which forms the broad overview from which a much more concretely oriented plan is derived. The mission statement itself may be very difficult to develop. The difficulty being compounded by different viewpoints, the lack of certainty of individual members of the committee and the possibility of the interaction of vested interest viewpoints as represented by different members of the planning body.

It is important that this process be carried out under the guidance of or with the assistance of a facilitator who can help the group work through what may be some very difficult moments. It is very easy to short-circuit this part of the process or even exclude it entirely. But very often the success or failure of the total plan rests in this first, somewhat arduous phase.

Some groups are so single-minded and tightly controlled that this component may not seem important. I assure you, however, that it is imperative it takes place, in great depth, even in the most tightly focused and controlled organization.

Once this identity is developed and accepted by consent, and the mission statement is developed and accepted and signed off by the members of the committee, then the roles and responsibilities of the committee and its constituent members can be further defined.

The definition of the roles that each individual member plays and their personal responsibility must be developed at the outset, even though there may not be specific assignments given. The definitions of these roles and responsibilities will allow for subsequent assignments of greater specificity as the process develops.

Some of these identity problems also include the size and composition of the group, time expenditures and meeting schedules. Additionally, the specific inclusion or exclusion of other individuals that may, at different points in time, be consultants, ex-officio or ad hoc members of the group will be necessary. The committee should also determine whether it will go through the development and construction phase, monitor the project, and be responsible for the evaluation and change. If not, who will perform these functions?

While all of these levels of identity may not be easily determined at the beginning, it is important that the issue be recognized early on. As the project continues, further clarification of these responsibilities in the different phases can be made. The strengths and weaknesses of the group must be assessed also. For example, if the primary purpose of the group is to fundraise in the community and members in this group have neither experience nor interest in fund-raising, the appropriateness of the group's makeup should be challenged. If a primary function of this group is to oversee construction and implementation, there should be members aboard who have had this type of experience.

Some planning processes factor in, at the outset, the need for two or more committees that function in an integrated fashion at different phases of the operation. There also may be sub-committees that pull in experts and consultants in different phases of the process. The committee should decide on its own internal operating procedure; who is the chair, who is the alternate chair, what rules do they follow when in session, what minimum vote do they need to support any particular issue, what is their relationship, if any, to existing corporate structures.

The next step in the identity phase is to develop the planning process in all of the ensuing steps, and have it approved in principle by the planning body. Included in this acceptance of the draft plan would be a rough outline of what is to be done, decisions to be made, and the time-lines that will add structure to the process. It is also appropriate, at this time, to assign specific responsibilities to individuals based on previously-determined roles.

ADMINISTRATOR'S RESPONSIBILITY

Since this is a textbook on administration, we must define the administrator's role in the planning process. It would be easy to say that the administrator's role is self-defined by that individual's education and experience. Certainly a person that has been through successful planning processes would have a different role than one who had no experience in that area. It is important, not from the administrator's standpoint, but from the planning committee's standpoint, to be able to assess the administrator's involvement with past planning processes and evaluate the success of that implementation. The assumption that an administrator, by virtue of having been involved in a planning process, is now expert enough to have a higher level of leadership is incorrect, unless confirmed by checking back on the success of that involvement.

Another factor that enters into the definition of the administrator's role is the size of the organization. The smaller the organization, the more difficult it is for an administrator to pull himself from operation and become involved in the broader overviews (and time commitment) required by the planning process. The larger the organization is, the greater the possibility that an associate or a subordinate level administrator will temporarily be given greater responsibility. An administrator simply cannot perform his full range of administrative duties *and* be a fully involved member of the planning process. Something has to "give." Before an administrator takes full responsibility, he must be able to get rid of his day-to-day operational tasks. If this cannot be accomplished, the responsibility of an administrator in the planning process must be somewhat subordinate to an external expert who comes in to supply the leadership and guidance needed to make the project successful.

When the administrator is the director of the total process, it must be assumed that there is a substantial experiential base to support this role, and that he can delegate the day-to-day operations to someone else. It is an uncommon administrator that finds himself in this situation.

The administrator has a very important role in bringing together the resources needed to make the planning process work (i.e., the people who form the body of the planning group, and the experts who input into the planning process). He must also be able to arrange for the fiscal needs of the planning process, because time and money are involved. Whether this be through a grant, funding from a parent organization, or funding from existing operations, the responsibility to have a firm economic base to the planning process itself is his alone.

The administrator, in some cases, may only play the role as a strategist or tactitian in terms of the program and implementation phase. In cases where outside consultants are called in to lead the planning process, the administrator's talents are pivotal to the success of the implementation and evaluation phase. In some cases the administrator must function as an educator, bringing his professional experience to the planning committee. He must serve as a motivator and agent of change to apprise the committee of trends and significant issues in the field of aging and long term care. An administrator who is professionally active will also be able to link the planning body with community, governmental, or professional organizations that will be able to support the planning process in a variety of necessary ways.

In those situations where the administrator is the person responsible for the total planning process, and not just another member of the team, there should be assurance that the administrator will stay through the evaluation and change phase. The mandate for a specific time commitment will place a greater emphasis on the administrator's long term role. The reverse, unfortunately, is the most common practice; that is, the leadership be it the administrator or an outside consultant is rarely responsible for monitoring the evaluation and change for the whole project. It is most common to find that the individuals who lead the planning process are not around during the implementation phase when all the problems usually develop. In a human service organization we see planners, be it the administrator or a professional planner, usually gone from the scene after the plan is developed and rarely around to take responsibility for any problems that arise during the implementation phase.

MARKET ANALYSIS PHASE

A marketing program is as much a necessity for a strategic plan as it is for the normal operation of a service. The more complete the plan is, the more accurate the project model phase will be, and the more successful will be the implementation. Modern technology contributes a great deal to the effective market plan. This should include, among other things: (a) an analysis of the area, including state, county, city and even neighborhood levels; (b) an analysis of existing facilities and services; (c) a demographic study of the population to be served including population trends, if possible, and the relationship between the state, county, city and local demographic factors; (d) service need indicators; (e) methods to access the population you are concerned with; (f) referral sources and pathways; (g) in-depth fiscal analysis of the demographics including income, ownership, family structure, etc.; (h) a promotional component that can design ways of reaching the appropriate consumer service or referral body. This "advertisement" and promotional component, often considered a marketing plan, is really just a component of the total program (marketing is discussed elsewhere in this text).

To continue with the marketing analysis, the expectations of major outside groups should be reviewed and analyzed as well as the major expectations of the sponsoring group. With this information we will have some good indicators of the interest of the community, as well as a greater understanding of the depth of interest of the constituent group sponsoring the plan.

PROJECT MODEL PHASE

This phase essentially describes just what you want to do. Will it be the creation of a physical plant, a nursing home, senior housing, home for the aged or board and care facility, or will it be the development of non brick and mortar programming? Here the market analysis will be used to guide the planning process to determine the best way to meet the needs of the user of services.

If, for example, a major thrust will be a brick and mortar facility, the exact services that this facility must deliver should be very clearly defined in terms of staffing, administrative policies, procedures and functions, and most importantly how it relates to the needs and wants of the user group. Here again it is very important to make a distinction between needs and wants, because each of these has a different value in terms of program development. Certainly, if an individual wants something, it is not necessarily the same as if he needs something. Often dialogues in planning sessions will spend a great deal of time trying to separate these two very different subjective terms.

FISCAL ANALYSIS PHASE

The fiscal analysis includes a thorough economic feasibility, current operational budget, and a projected three year operational budget for the sake of completeness.

The feasibility study should define, in great detail, the expenses that will be incurred through the implementation phase, including planning, development, construction, and so forth. It should also very clearly delineate income sources and develop a bottom line indicating profit, breakeven or loss. In the case of many nonprofit organizations, the deficit that occurs is made up through other sources, usually within the constituent population that it serves. Ongoing economic feasibilities and capital development have been discussed in other chapters.

If correctly done, the feasibility study will create a variety of options, mixing and matching combinations of income sources, census levels, patient mix by payor, and reimbursement trends.

An additional component of this economic feasibility would be the description of sources of funding, i.e., HUD funding for senior housing, FHA funding for nursing home construction, private bank funding, health authority funding, bond issue development, etc. If a community-wide fund-raising drive, or a fund-raising drive within the constituent group is intended, then that project should be defined, and a separate fund-raising effort initiated from this component of the planning phase.

PROCEDURAL PROCESSING PHASE

While the project model phase may consist of recommendations that relate to two or more services or structures being developed within contiguous timelines, the procedural processing phase will include the wide variety of approvals that will be needed to get the project off and running. It should include acquiring appropriate legal advice, include local or regional planning permits, and a certificate of need, if necessary. It may include an environmental impact study, sale testings, zoning restriction, planning waivers, etc. These procedural steps should be designed in a very tight time frame with clear assignments for all parties concerned. Here again the use of consultants, attorneys or advisors of all kinds requires a great deal of coordination and planning. There are many pieces of paper flowing back and forth, and a great deal of energy must be put forth so that these various procedural steps are accomplished in the shortest period of time.

Just applying for a certificate of need, if that is required, or a zoning change, may take the better part of a year. The more tightly managed this process is the shorter the total planning program will be. Some of these steps may be totally thwarted by a variety of approval agencies, and may require waivers, and even court action to break through bureaucratic barriers. In some cases, as with certificates of need, community support is needed. Here's where information about the community is important, because support groups within the community can be of great assistance in helping you get a variety of approvals needed to get the project off the ground.

DESIGN AND DEVELOPMENT PHASE

The design and development is a translation of the project model phase into actual building design, construction specifications, and space allocations. The design and development phase usually requires the involvement of an architect, if one is not already on the planning committee, and a consultant who is particularly knowledgeable about the actual design requirement of the project being planned. Sometimes the committee's architect brings this skill and competency with him, other times an architect with specialized knowledge must be brought in. This design and development phase should include details of the space each program will need; location of people, equipment and functions; schematic drawings representing all of these; and be tied in to cost estimates for different phases of this design process. It would be very good if the total design and development phase could be presented in a schematic or pert chart showing the serial steps that must be accomplished for the completion of the project. There should be an agreed procedure for reviewing the preliminary drawings, and there should be sign off procedure by the planning committee and the sponsoring body that, in essence, says the plans have been approved or modified acceptably. Signing off consensus opinions is vitally important for maintaining continuity, assuring buy-in and refreshing everyone's memory as time goes on and details become obscure. Signing off on drawings is just one of the many approaches to pursuing this strategic plan. It is also advisable during the design and development phase to address the aesthetics of the environment being created by pulling in viewpoints in addition to those of the professionals involved. One of the most unsuccessful elements of strategic planning has been the reliance solely on professional input in addressing aesthetic components of work and service delivery space.

Serious consideration should be given in determining who the reviewing bodies will be. Certainly, if this a community nonprofit organization, select individuals who are part of constituency or governance of the organization would logically be part of the review of the design of the project. Secondly, since the ultimate acceptance of the project is based on the perceptions of staff and user (i.e., client or patient) the viewpoint of these parties will be vital. It is unlikely that there will be a total agreement on the part of all concerned, but many projects have failed because they did not take into account constructive criticism from those who actually use the space. At this point, I would like to re-emphasize that the administrator must define his role in each phase of the planning process. Because of the misconception of his level of authority or control over the project, the administrator is often put in an untenable position. His level of actual authority and control over the project may vary as each different phase is entered upon. It is the astute administrator that recognizes this fact. Because very often the burden of a failed project is laid on the desk of the administrator, it is important not to take anything for granted. Not only, therefore, must sign offs (representing buy-ins) become a routine part of the entire ten-stage process, but the definition of the role and responsibility of the administrator must be clear at every stage.

Consultants (architectural firms, fiscal specialists or contractors) reduce the cost of acquiring specialized knowledge. Without them, the learning curve for bringing in technical support to the committee would be lengthy and costly. There are few architectural firms, for example, who have extensive experience in this particular field; yet many firms will be more than willing to attempt this project and learn at your expense.

Another very important reason for the checking and double checking the design is the real problem of taking corrective action once the contracts for construction are signed. The need for construction change orders has arisen time and again, not necessarily due to tight specs being found in error, but to major functional changes that do not become evident until contracts are signed and the project is well underway. Change orders are very costly and must be reduced to a minimum. The best way to reduce this is with heavily loading front end analysis of the project design with as many different viewpoints as is possible. This "front end" emphasis on the approval of design will be very profitable in the long run.

Sometimes projects are moving along so quickly that they develop a head of steam at the time that project design review takes place. If this project is moving so swiftly that it cannot be controlled to allow for these approvals, the administrator must document his position quite clearly so that his responsibility of pointing out the need for this level of review is part of the record of the project.

A valid part of project design is actually taking the time for select members of the project group to see comparable facilities. Money invested in travel and observation and dialogue is well spent and adds to the understanding of the functional as well as the aesthetic value of the project. At all times, the social and psychological needs of the *users* of the service, whether client, resident, or patient must be considered. Their movement patterns during the day must be given at least as much value as the functional use of the space for efficient staff purposes. Design should include current concepts of environmental queueing that have been developed and implemented successfully. This goes beyond signage or a merely directional approach to guiding people through the environment; it should incorporate use of color, shape, texture and other elements that will not only enhance the environment from a living standpoint, but will be quite utilitarian in helping people to get from one point to another.

While the following points were probably addressed during the project model phase, they should be reconsidered in the light of the model design. Elements of the psychosocial need of the occupants should be explored in great depth to assure that the space offers options for movement, reasonable privacy, and has communality capabilities. Space design should encourage not isolation, but social interaction, independence and enhancement of self-esteem.

The design feature that has raised a great deal of concern recently is the utilization of larger open wards for the more debilitated patients. The large open ward is, in my opinion, an excellent social milieu for caring for the older, more disabled patient. It helps to prevent loneliness and isolation and if handled properly, can be developed into a small community or supportive social nucleus that will add to the stimulation of daily living. The open wards, while appearing to some to be a throwback to former physical designs, may be a totally appropriate and healthy environment for a large number of the people now entering the long-term care system at the institutional level.

CONSTRUCTION PHASE

The next phase is the construction phase. In many cases, the administrator is out of the picture during the construction phase. Whether the project is brand new or an addition to an existing plan, the emphasis during construction often puts architect and contractor in roles that minimize the need for administrative involvement. It is the responsibility of the administrator, however, to clearly define their responsibilities during the construction phase (as he has during other phases). Depending on the administrator's level in the overall project, he will need to manage the communication between the architect and construction firm, and the governing body and project committee. This means passing on successful completion of various goals in the construction project; problems connected with change orders, and any problems whose magnitude may obstruct the successful completion of the project. It is very important to have absolutely clear the relationship between architect and contractor and understand completely who is responsible for insuring that the contractor follows all the specifics required of him. Ambiguity in this role of architect-contractor relationship will cause problems. By and large it is the professional role of the architect to insure that his plans are being followed, but nevertheless, the administrator must make his presence felt during the process in order to guarantee success of the total project.

These construction programs often impact the neighborhood, the community or the existing physical plant. The administrator must play a role in resolving any problems that arise, and therefore must maintain a presence close enough to the construction project to respond to neighborhood, community, or workforce problems before they get out of hand.

IMPLEMENTATION

The implementation phase must begin well in advance of the actual date the doors to the plant open. A plan for hiring of appropriate staff must be developed at least a year prior to the opening date to leave time for recruitment of personnel. The timed recruitment plan must coincide with the availability of funding and take into account an anticipated admission of maximum census. Most nursing homes in the current marketplace will fill quite quickly, therefore, it is appropriate to have a majority of the operating staff on hand at (or near) the opening date. Types of housing, such as retirement housing, may take months to fill up and, in these cases, the recruitment plan should take into account a slower employment of new hires until complete maximum census is reached.

The marketing plan, which should have a phase specifically directed at opening and promoting the new service, should also be timed well in advance. Many such plans attempt to develop a waiting list in order to shorten the timeline for filling the facility. In the case of life care or continuing care it is common to promote a service facility up to a year in advance. This advanced marketing approach is advantageous not only to the facility, but to seniors who are given a longer timeline to plan the social and physical transitions that will take place.

The development of operational policy and procedure and the establishment of optimal departmental effectiveness can only take place with a great deal of front-end planning. All the policies and procedures and systems (business, food service, etc.) should be developed in advance, and staff given the opportunity to be trained in their use before the facility opens. If development of staff familiarity with operational procedure is delayed until after the doors open, confusion is bound to result. This altogether-too-common practice not only creates an unstable administration, but very often has direct consequences on cash flow, revenue projections, and fiscal stability in general.

MONITORING

Once the construction is completed and the implementation of the use of the physical plant is begun, a very close monitoring program must be started. The nature and format of this monitoring program will, of course, be specified periods of time. The monitoring plan should have a specialized team of people (hopefully some that were connected with the plan from the start) review planned key points and develop a method of reporting and presenting them. While the planned monitoring of the physical plant design may be of relatively short duration, that component of the plan that checks operations within the facility may become an ongoing quality assurance program. In any event, the monitoring process is in the form of an audit and should be as quantifiable as possible. The monitoring body (or person) may or may not evaluate its own findings—which brings us to the next and final step in our process and one that is very important.

EVALUATION AND CHANGE

If the monitoring program shows up flaws in the basic space design, what good does it do to point these out? At the stage of the monitoring step what can you do to change the brick and mortar? The walls are up, the building is occupied; your options are limited—yes, but not excluded. If the monitoring program points out problems with the space during its evaluation period, you may find that the space problem is really one of function. It is important to understand this. It may be that staff has not had the proper education in the use of the space. It may be that new functions are taking place, and people are unfamiliar with them. It may be that the internal system is incorrect. There are a variety of problems with physical plants that do not entail actually changing the structural integrity of the building, but point to education, new systems and perhaps a reallocation of resources. If the evaluation of the space points to actual physical plant flaws, there is *still* opportunity, in the short run, to redesign (on a limited basis) structural components of the building. The primary variable here is the availability of additional funds to do so. Certainly, if the space problems are the fault of the contractor, or even the fault of errors in architectural design, the contractor or architect should assume the responsibility for making the necessary plant changes.

Let's say, however, that the monitoring, when evaluated, shows up flaws in areas other than the physical plant per se. For example, what if the furnishings are inadequate or incorrect? What if the rules of the organization are too restrictive or too lenient to allow successful delivery of services? What if certain functions, such as recreation, kitchen or dining facilities and health-oriented services do not have adequate space, equipment or functional design? It could be the population that has become resident in the project turns out not to have the same profile as that population that was projected as coming into the project. So we find that what must happen is not necessarily physical plan change, but change related to internal operational programming. Most of these changes will relate to basic living situations, and not to complex program delivery. They will relate to the needs of the occupants in terms of daily living: the freedom of access to various parts of the building; the availability to meet in privacy with family and friends; the availability of appropriate, health-oriented services (if they are a part of the project) and they will relate to noticeable problems with aesthetics and ambiance of the environment. Many of these difficulties can be readily improved upon.

Very often the subjective feelings of the patient or resident are the prime determinants of the success of program implementation. When evaluated, they will point out ways various living systems can be easily altered. It is important to listen to the subjective viewpoints of the staff and the occupant and respond very quickly to their suggestions. It may even be important to have these critiques done jointly, so that the solutions will be acceptable to all parties.

Problems to do with safety features, private kitchen availability, examining areas, etc., will directly affect the long term success of the project. It is important to address these issues and make changes as soon as possible. Recognize, also, that once the first phase of the evaluation and change take place, it only indicates that the monitoring function must kick in. Monitoring, evaluation and change must be intensive during the first six months of operation. When the project stabilizes, and most of the corrective actions have taken place and are successful, the astute administrator will implement such monitoring, evaluation and change processes on a planned basis throughout the years. It is inevitable that changes will be needed and it is much better to pick them up in an organized fashion as part of a routine administrative process. Otherwise internal disputes, conflicts and user dissatisfaction will come to the attention of the administrator when the problems have reached a critical level.

Financing of the
Long Term Care System

We will deal with financing of the long term care system from two viewpoints. First of all, we will deal with the capital formation system, and secondly we will deal with the operating revenue sources.

CAPITAL FUNDING OF LONG TERM CARE SYSTEM

Capital funding of long term care primarily addresses the fiscal needs encountered when creating a physical plant to deliver a service; that is the construction of senior housing, residential, skilled nursing, or some combination of these levels of care. We will not address the start-up costs of a delivery system, which many people view as part of the capital funding program. Certainly we must recognize that to begin any service system, whether it be an adult day health care, a nutrition site, or home health agency, physical plant is a requisite. The important aspect to these programs, however, may not be physical plant per se, but start-up costs or seed money, which are viewed by some people as capital in nature. It should be pointed out that the primary mechanisms are through certain specific seed money funds within Housing and Urban Development, special foundation grants, and privately financed bank loans.

Seed Money

Housing and Urban Development (HUD) has a program to provide interest-free seed money loans to nonprofit sponsors for the purpose of stimulating low and moderate income housing. This program (called Section 106B) is available through application to HUD. The Housing Assistance Council is a nonprofit corporation which offers seed money for rural low income people. It is primarily for use by public, private or nonprofit organizations in the construction or rehabilitation of housing for these low income rural families. Many states have housing finance agencies which offer interest-free loans to get projects off the ground. Since these are statutory, each state must be contacted and an inquiry made.

Private Foundations

Since many nonprofit sponsors have been recipients of grants from private foundations, we must recognize that this may be their only source of seed money. The process of seeking money from private foundations is an art unto itself and very often it is advisable to seek professional help to access the foundation funding sources.

Fund drives or special donations are very often the quickest route to acquiring seed money. Usually there are fewer regulatory strings attached to funds acquired in this fashion and used in the proper manner.

Various configurations of equity syndication utilize existing tax laws to make contributions advantageous to individuals. These are often successful vehicles to acquire seed money and may be utilized in conjunction with some of the other efforts mentioned earlier.

When creating of these start-up funds there must be adequate attention paid to the need for float to allow the organization to survive until projected income starts to materialize. Recognition must be given to the long periods of time between the start-up of any particular program and the potential receipts of income especially if they are government funded programs. The relationship between start-up costs and float must be thoroughly thought out if the organization is to survive during the first few months of its operation. Many an agency has folded because of improperly calculating the income cash flow and not having adequate monies in reserve to use as float until this income is realized.

Capital Funding Options

There are three primary vehicles for the funding of capital construction: (1) conventional mortgage loans; (2) FHA programs; and (3) revenue bonds. Private and public sectors utilize these vehicles in different manners.

Private Financing Mechanisms

When we refer to private financing we automatically, by definition, exclude funds received from governmental sources. These non-governmental sources would include any of the following, and sometimes combinations of more than one: public taxable bonds, tax exempt revenue bonds, housing finance agencies on a state level, taxable bonds privately placed, gifts, bequests or endowments, founders' fees, conventional mortgage loans and admission or entry fees.

Conventional Mortgage Loans

This is not unlike financing for an individual's home. Most commonly used are savings and loan associations, banks, life insurance companies and pension funds.

Taxable Bonds—Privately Placed

Under these circumstances, an investment banking firm or industrial bond house underwrites a loan and distributes bonds to private investors, such as pension funds, etc. The underwriter charges a fee, usually taken in a form of a discount when the bonds are issued.

Revenue Bonds—Tax Exempt

Because states have allowed the promulgation of this practice, many organizations have found this a good vehicle because the interest on these bonds is exempt from federal taxes. Because of this, investors are normally willing to accept a slightly lower return on their investment. These bonds may be issued by a state or municipal government hospital or health authority or by a city or even by a large credible nonprofit corporation.

Gifts

This is of major importance to nonprofit groups who have a constituency. It is very common for them to raise equity or seed money through the method of fund solicitation. The art of fund-raising from both constituency groups and the community at large is a talent and skill that many successful administrators have.

Entry Fee

There are a variety of types of entry fees, sometimes labeled founders' fees or admission fees. Very often these contributions buy a certain package of services as well as the possibility of some form of equity in the physical plant itself. Concomitant with these entry fees are often a variety of covenants that restrict the use of these entry fees. Most states which allow this activity have very sophisticated methods of auditing and protecting the rights of the admittee so that the use of these entry fees are as agreed upon on admission.

Housing Finance Agencies as Part of State Government

These agencies are statutory in nature and not only provide funding, but often couple this with technical assistance for the less sophisticated sponsor. The types of financing usually funded are construction or permanent financing and seed money at low or interest-free rates.

Taxable Bonds, Public Sector

This is the most widely utilized method of financing hospitals, and it is currently a major alternative for funding physical plant construction in the long term care field. These public taxable bonds have very strict guidelines for their use and usually require expert consultation to develop and implement the funding package.

Miscellaneous Methods

Funding often requires a patchwork of two or more techniques to get the desired money to allow for construction and operation of the program. Because of the very positive impact a long term care facility will have in the community, unsecured notes may be tendered by local financing agencies who are interested in this broader impact of the long term care facility on the community.

PUBLIC FINANCING

This, in essence, is the utilization of federal government money for physical plant projects in long term care. Under this we have four major vehicles: Housing and Urban Development (HUD), Veteran's Administration, Department of Health and Human Service, and Farmers Home Administration.

Housing and Urban Development (HUD)

The U.S. Department of Housing and Urban Development, known as HUD, was established in 1965 a generation after the implementation of the National Housing Act of 1934. The primary agency within HUD that is able to create numerous loan and mortgage insurance packages is the Federal Housing Administration (FHA).

Some of the more common funding vehicles that are used under the FHA auspices are the following sections: cooperative housing . . . section 213, urban renewal development . . . section 220, market interest rates . . . section 221D, 3 and 4, elderly housing . . . section 231 nursing homes . . . section 232, condominiums . . . 234, rental housing and interest subsidy . . . section 236, and hospitals . . . 242.

Section 101, rent supplements support low income persons living in privately owned and operated multi-family projects whose mortgages were insured under certain HUD programs.

Section 119 is an urban development action grant that is designed to assist cities and urban counties to gentrify neighborhoods. They most normally work to establish a partnership between government and the private sector. Although this type of funding for long term care facilities may be viewed as not related to the duties of the average administrator, it is quite conceivable that a professionally active administrator would become part of this city-wide or area-wide program and, therefore, be able to lend his expertise in management to the construction of appropriate long term care facilities under Section 119.

Section 202 were direct loans for housing elderly and handicapped, primarily granted to nonprofit sponsors. This funding also included the rehabilitation of housing for the elderly or handicapped and has historically included congregate housing for the elderly as described in a previous chapter. Restoring 202 funding levels has been a major goal of organizations active in the senior housing field.

Section 213 is federal insurance for loans made by private lending institutions to finance co-op housing. The sponsor must either be a nonprofit corporation or have the intent to sell the cooperative to a nonprofit corporation or trust.

Section 220 are thoroughly insured loans which will finance mortgages in housing and designated urban renewal areas.

Sections 221 (D,3) and 221 (D,4) provide mortgage insurance for rental housing and co-ops for low and moderate income families.

Section 231 was established by the National Housing Act of 1959 with the intent of providing adequate housing to meet the needs of the elderly and the handicapped. Here the federal government offers mortgage insurance to aid the development of new or substantially rehabilitated rental housing for elderly or handicapped individuals and their families.

Section 232 provides federal mortgage insurance for financing of construction and/or rehabilitation and nursing or intermediate care facilities. Sponsors in this case may either be a nonprofit or proprietary corporation. Section 232 is a federal insurance program to finance the construction or rehabilitation of condominium projects that were built under the Section 232 of the National Housing Act.

Section 236 provides assistance to sponsors in the development and operation of housing for low income personnel by insuring loans from private sector financial institutions.

Section 241 enables multi-family housing projects, nursing homes, intermediate care facilities, hospitals and other institutions to finance necessary improvements and additions to their projects. It may also be used to purchase equipment and furniture for nursing homes and related facilities. The financing can be used to supplement existing mortgages and can be made available without refinancing existing mortgages. Section 241 provides federal mortgage insurance to finance the construction or rehabilitation of nonprofit or profit motivated hospitals. Proprietary and nonprofit organizations have access to these funds.

Farmers Home Administration Program

This is actually a division of the Department of Agriculture and has several programs that can be used for housing for the elderly. These may either be direct loans or guaranteed loans through a lender or sponsor.

Under Section 306 of the Farmers Home Administration there are funds through the community facilities loan program that are available to agencies and nonprofit associations for the purpose of constructing, enlarging and improving community facilities in urban areas. These may include senior centers, health clinics, community centers, etc.

Section 515 of the Farmers Home Administration allows for rural rental housing loans for multi-family rental projects. This relates to both subsidized and unsubsidized loans for these multi-family projects.

Health and Human Service

Under Title V of the Old Americans Act, as amended in 1975, there is some funding available for senior centers.

Veterans Administration

The Veterans Administration may make grants of up to 65% of the project's costs with the balance being picked up by the sponsoring state. The sponsorship is limited only to state governmental agencies, who direct their efforts to eligible veterans in that state.

FINANCING OF OPERATIONAL NEEDS

Since this text is primarily for administrators of long term care facilities, we will view financing of long term service as it relates to the requisites of managing a facility or service. Very often, in the published material on financing for long term care, the concern primarily is on the macrovision and national public policy. The financial level we are describing, however, is that which must be totally understood by the administrator in order for the successful accomplishment of their organizational goals.

The individual who receives long term care services must either pay privately or be eligible for governmentally supported programs. For example, about 55% of nursing home costs are now paid by federal and state contributions.

Medicare

The Medicare program initially widely believed to be the primary long term health support system for the elderly, is almost exclusively directed for services rendered in the acute hospital. The most rapidly growing component of the Medicare system is the home health agency expenditures, which currently cover about 18% of the Medicare program. The recently implemented diagnostic related group system (DRG) has prematurely discharged patients to skilled nursing or their homes. Added home health services will be needed to care for this sicker population at home, whether it was created by the DRG process or is the result of the existence of an older and sicker group of elderly people.

The economic instability of the Medicare hospital insurance trust fund indicates that there will be continued pressure to expand the use of services perceived to be less costly. The long term consequences of this practice increased recidivism back to the acute hospital.

Medicaid Program

Title XIX of the Social Security Acts provides for a medical assistance program for certain low income individuals and families. Medicaid, as the program is known, became law in 1965. It followed the Kerr-Mills program of medical assistance for the aging.

Medicaid program is the primary funding for the long term care system. Over 40% of Medicaid program benefits are directed towards the long term care. Medicaid also provides federal matching grants to states for operating health financing programs for low income persons. The federal matching share ranges from 50% to 75% depending on a negotiated rate between the federal government and the states. The primary categories supported by the Medicaid program are aged, blind and disabled, and families with dependent children. Medicaid's substantial growth in the recent past has been augmented by the shift of residents by state mental hospitals to community-based long term care programs. This movement of mental health dischargees into the local long term care system has been assisted by supplemental security income assistance, food stamps and housing aids. In certain parts of the county intermediate care facilities have become the primary care site for mentally retarded dischargees from state hospitals.

Although all trends seem to predict an expansion of the needs for long term care services, federal and state governments as well as private insurers have not expanded benefits substantially because of their concern for the uncontrolled potential service demand.

Additional to the potential increase in service demand is the possibility that many services now provided by relatives may no longer be provided by them if comparable services are federally funded. Please remember, the majority of frail elderly are supported by an informal network of friends, families and neighbors. This fragile informal network could be seriously impacted by the augmentation of existing formal support systems.

The following is the list of services commonly covered by the Medicaid program:

1. inpatient hospital services
2. outpatient hospital services
3. laboratory and x-ray
4. skilled nursing
5. home health services
6. intermediate care services
7. physician services
8. family planning service
9. rural health clinic services
10. mid-wife services
11. early periodic screening and diagnosis for certain classes of clients.

States may add to this basic service pattern if they wish. They may also determine the scope of services offered.

Medicare/Medicaid Relationship

Many people are covered by both Medicaid and Medicare programs. When individuals are eligible for both of these programs, Medicare will make the primary payment for the service and the state Medicaid expenditure is, therefore, limited to the deductible and copayment amounts that are part of the total reimbursement formula. The line of demarcation that distinguishes where one program pays and the other picks up the costs is often a point of contention between the two funding vehicles. The many interrelationships between the state and federal aspects of Medicaid and the state Medicaid administration and the federal Medicare programs is beyond the scope of this text. Suffice to say, that it is imperative that this relationship be understood thoroughly by the administrator, recognizing that as part of the interplay one program may seek to cut its costs by shifting costs onto the other program. Understanding this interplay and being able to "manage it" will increase the effectiveness of the administrator in dealing with this substantial income source.

LONG TERM CARE INSURANCE

Everyone is concerned about the devastating impact that the cost of long-term care has on the elderly population. Countless stories are made public about life savings being totally exhausted by relatively short periods of stay in skilled nursing facilities. There is also great concern on the part of government on how to fund future long-term care costs, particularly with the radical increase in the over 75 population and concurrent increase in degrees of medical acuity of their health problems. Whether or not there should be long-term care insurance should no longer be debated. The policy questions, rather, should related to the market development, the nature of coverage provisions, and the relationship of private market to public programs.

Market Development

Most of the focus has been on developing a marketable package of benefits that make fiscal sense to a private sector insurance company. The marketability of this package depends on many factors, one of which is the attitude of seniors themselves. While many do not think they will need LTC insurance, or overestimate the value of their existing coverage (i.e., with a MediGap type of insurance). The author feels that the level of consciousness of seniors is much higher than previously thought.

Defining the marketplace would also reflect on the ability of families of older people to pay premiums as well as younger people who have the opportunity for long range financial planning. As a market incentive, current tax benefits through deductions and credits may be a successful lure for children with older parents.

This expanded marketing approach would spread the risk more broadly and enhance the economic feasibility. Efforts to test market this broad based participation should be accelerated.

Early on, policy discussions should address the LTC insurance needs of non-elderly disabled and veterans. How would their inclusion/exclusion shape the market of potential participants?

Could inclusion of LTC insurance in existing retirement plans be a way of expanding the base of premium payments?

Should special attention be given to test marketing of LTC insurance plans specifically related to home health and adult day care?

Benefit Package

Perhaps the real debate will center on the very complex issue of benefit packages. It is not enough to say the LTC insurance should cover services of the continuum, both institutional and non-institutional. Initially, key services should be targeted, that is SNF, ICF, Adult Day Care and Home Care. The industry's concern about defining non-institutional benefits in a way that will not induce demand must be addressed. If there is an increase in demand for benefits it may be a reflection of needs currently not being met.

Another controversial component of insurance plans are complex utilization controls, such as:

1. pre-existing condition limits
2. prior hospitalization requirements
3. medical screening and physical exams
4. restrictions on mental, drugs, and alcohol conditions
5. restrictive definitions of coverage and service
6. elimination periods

In my observation, one of the most difficult aspects is the determination of the insurability of what is commonly called "custodial type care." I suggest this because the insurance industry is currently tooled up to deal with medical and medically related problems. Thus far activities of daily living including bathing, dressing, feeding, companionship and social support services have not been configured in the scope of current insurance coverage. While there is every reason to believe that effect insurance coverage for home care, adult day health care and similar non-institutional services would ultimately be both profitable to the insurer and cost-effective to the system as a whole in the long run, more test of benefit packages should be made.

We should also be concerned about benefit packages that exclude chronic conditions associated with normal aging. An area of potential problems is the need for better assessment devices to assess type and level of care, for people who have many physical problems often accompanied by mental impairment.

Private Market and Public Programs

During the last decade, when talk of long-term care insurance evolved from rhetoric into hardcore legislation, there has been little, if any, dialogue concerning the impact of these insurance concepts on the medically indigent population that is served by the local public sector. In the last couple of years, public sector long-term care has taken on a new meaning by virtue of the inclusion in the public sector responsibility of adult day health care, home care and other components of the continuum that heretofore have been exclusively in the domain of the private sector.

The state's assistance in the creation of a proprietary insurance vehicle could significantly leverage the use of public funds, both state and local. To be more specific, exposure of the government to LTC costs will be reduced to the extent that Medicaid is deferred. Long-term care insurance should not be thought of as a substitute for Medicaid, but as an additional option to choose from. Concurrently, the private insurance marketplace would increase consumers choice and expand the diversification of services concurrently available.

This form of cost shifting would be reflected by the degree to which the premiums paid by the recipient forms the pool of money paid to the providers of care. In terms of the utilization of the pool of funds available to pay providers, the elderly community will be most interested in utilization standards and the role of whoever is assumed to be the gatekeeper for the rendering of services. It would be unfortunate if utilization standards would be more complex than they are currently for Medicaid and Medicare. Without addressing complex issues such as creation of a high risk pool (to insure carriers for problems of adverse selection) with the state as a conduit for these funds, we must consider both the economic and social implications of any percentage of the primary Medicaid population having adjunct insurance that pays for all or part of their care.

To the extent that these and many other questions are rhetorical, state governments have an opportunity to begin a serious dialogue by the establishment of task forces of providers of care, providers of insurance and consumers that will respond to these and many other questions in an intelligent and planned way.

The utopian solution would be one that benefited the seniors, brought profits to the insurance carrier and allowed the state to have greater control over the tax dollars needed to support the system.

Public Policy

The discussion of public policy in long term care could be the most complex part of this textbook. Probably the most difficult aspect is the presentation of information on public policy that has some relativity to the functioning of the administrator of a long term care facility or service. This abstracting of appropriate public policy material is complicated by the remoteness of public policy formulation from the delivery of service. The tremendous schism between public policy planners and practitioners is in itself a major barrier to both the successful development and implementation of public policy. In this chapter we will attempt to deal with the subject of public policy as it relates to the practitioner; that is, how administrators can be part of public policy development and interpret public policy in a manner that will allow them both to effectively run their organizations and appropriately plan for its future activities. In this chapter we address public policy both at the federal and state level, recognizing at the outset that public policy is a coalescence of views and opinions from a variety of governmental and non-governmental sources. Public policies are those policies which enacted legislation reflects as law. Administrative interpretation of this law frequently is construed to be public policy and may or may not be consistent with the basic intent of the law. Action on the administrative level is itself public policy.

For many years people in the field of aging have been calling for a national public policy on aging and long term care. There seems to be no resolution of this issue, even though there have been many laws enacted in the field of long term care. Most people feel that the lack of a national policy from the executive and legislative branch of this country in itself constitutes *de facto* policy. Consequently, where there exists an absence of policy, it is construed to be the intentional policy of *status quo*. This abstruse reasoning has dominated public policy in long term care for the last two decades. From the government's viewpoint, the requirement that public policy must be implemented has caused leadership to shy away from overcommitting in a field that is dynamically and rapidly changing. The piecemeal legislative approaches that appear to fight fires is apparently not only the way of the past but the way of the future as well.

Let's briefly review the historical development of public policy.

PUBLIC POLICY: HISTORICAL PERSPECTIVE

In 1950 President Truman directed that a national conference on aging be held to address various problems that were emerging as a result of the uncommon increase in numbers of elderly persons. Although there were no specific actions taken, a variety of recommendations were generated that became the first guidelines for national action. The problems increased in magnitude so that in 1958 Congress requested President Eisenhower to call a White House conference on aging which was held in January of 1961. The recommendations produced by this first White House Conference on Aging were implemented during the early '60s. And as we discussed in reviewing the history of long term care, Medicare and Medicaid were two of the public policy recommendations generated by the White House Conference which were implemented and which formed the basis for our current financial structuring of long term care. Additional to the Medicare/Medicaid Program, public policy that increased social security benefits was also developed. Dissatisfaction with the government programs designated to serve the elderly were a major factor in the passage of the Older American Act in 1965. The act which established the Administration on Aging as the federal focal point and the advocate for concerns of the nation's older person was designed to foster coordination and increase commitment of federal resources to the field of aging. Some programs were funded for research and demonstration in aging, and some for training manpower to serve older people. Public policy based on this White House Conference also addressed issues of housing, manpower training for older workers and new volunteer opportunities. All this being said, there still was no comprehensive set of national policies directing all levels and parts of the government in a cohesive manner.

Still, older people appeared to be disadvantaged with unacceptably high levels of poverty and with inflation continuing to undercut limited resources. In the late sixties, the Department of Health Education and Welfare was restructured and the Administration on Aging lost a large amount of program responsibilities. This was viewed as a major setback for the aging advocates. The ensuing second White House Conference on Aging called by President Nixon at the request of Congress was actually a three year process consisting of a prologue year (1970), a year designated as the year of conferences (1971), and the following year was projected as the year of action. The conference produced an incredible set of recommendations. The overriding goal of all of the recommendations was to assist the aging person to maintain his or her independence by assuring: (1) an adequate income; (2) appropriate living arrangements; (3) independence and dignity; and (4) institutional responsiveness and a new attitude towards aging.

While delegates to the 1971 White House Conference had often appeared critical of the administration's response to the conference's recommendation, there is substantial documentation to show that many laws were enacted as a direct result of this conference. During the decade that followed, a great many laws supporting non-institutional services and income stabilization for the elderly were enacted.

In 1974 the Federal Council on Aging was formed to address, at the highest level of public policy, the needs of the elderly. Of primary concern to the Council were the needs of the frail elderly which were viewed as elderly over 75 who needed an array of support services that could be offered by the continuum of care we have discussed. By 1977 there was a national network on aging in place consisting of 56 state agencies and 556 area agencies on aging. There were over 1000 nutrition agencies operating over 9000 sites providing both congregate and home delivered meals. Other services such as information and referral, telephone reassurance, chore services, in-home support services, escort services, and legal and other counseling services were initiated and funded through Title III of the Older American's Act.

The creation of an advocacy network for elderly needs began also in the early seventies as an off-shoot of the White House Conference. By 1979, the planning for the third White House Conference on Aging was initiated by President Carter. The change in governmental leadership to President Reagan engendered what was claimed to be partisan politics in structuring the conference, which, some alleged, influenced the outcome. Nevertheless, the project which took three years to complete produced over 650 individual recommendations for public policy actions.

This brief synopsis of public policy in retrospect leads us to current issues facing the government. Many of these issues are related to those highlighted by the 1981 White House Conference and some have been generated by major system changes that have taken place since the conference.

NATIONAL ISSUES

Any exploration of public policy on a national level must include recognition of the complexity of existing programs and their interrelations at the federal government level. There are many committees and agencies that have jurisdiction over different parts of long term care system. When one sees the explosion of interorganizational relationships on the Senate and House side of the legislative bodies, one can easily understand how the entire long term care system has defied significant public policy development. The obvious fragmentation is in itself a problem which hinders the development of consistent national long term care policies. The complexity demonstrated by this matrix fosters gaps and intrinsic conflicts in service delivery that could be unattended due to lack of any system oversight. It is believed also that this confounding series of relationships between program and legislative committees adds to the power of vested interest groups who make their wishes or demands known to one single element of this design and thereby prevent any broad range collective effort at coordination of proper resource allocation. There is also a high probability for overlap of service and efforts.

In this text we have dealt solely with the most predominant services in the long term care continuum and have not addressed the myriad of programs that exist for our elderly population. We have attempted to focus on primary services in the long term care continuum, but must recognize that a variety of other programs sponsored by the federal government may interrelate at different times. They most assuredly offer services above and beyond what may be considered in our discussion of long term care. Their very existence however makes public policy in the long term care arena much more difficult and makes the responsibility of the administrator that much greater if he is to be a well-informed practitioner in the field of long term care.

SYSTEM CHANGES

Thus far we have described public policy in a generic form. We will now address the extension of broad range public policy to include derivative changes within existing federal and state systems. It is very easy for an administrator to view the governing matrices of state and federal overview as impenetrable and static.

The idea that public policy is resistant to change is easy to accept when grappling with the frustrations of frontline administration. In reality, public policy is fluid and dynamic. At any one point in time, many issues that are cause for concern for the operating administrator will be undergoing important changes. Not only are many troublesome areas undergoing corrective change, but we are also able to specify channels through which the administrator may impact these changes.

THE ADMINISTRATOR AS A CHANGEMAKER

This section is not intended as a basic course for political activism nor does it intend to overwork the phrase "changemaker." What we shall attempt, however, is to describe some rather clear tracks the administrator has to access public policy on both the state and federal level. The most significant method for administrators to impact public policy is through the professional associations that operate within the long term care system. All major organizations have, at some point, contact with policy makers on a federal and state level. For example, the American Association of Homes for the Aging, the National Council on Aging, the American Healthcare Association, etc., all have very active public policy subsections. The administrators who choose to become involved at the grassroots level, and ultimately at regional and national levels, have an excellent opportunity to have their voice heard. This activity should be encouraged, since the best public policy in my opinion is that which originates from field-based viewpoints. The experienced frontline administrator can contribute more to successful public policy than any other one class of professionals.

Another way to become involved in public policy formulation is to work closely with advocacy groups or political action groups that may be more broad-based. For example, it is not impossible to be connected with the local political organization (party of your choice) and through this political vehicle make your voice heard. It is not unusual for administrators to have personal contact with congresspersons or state legislators and find that they can access public policy by establishing rapport over the years with these political leaders. When dealing with congresspersons or state legislators, it is important to make contact with their key staff personnel, since the staff rather than the legislator will be your primary contact.

These kinds of contacts, both professional and political, take tremendous amounts of time. Most of these relationships must be built up over the long haul, and will require a great deal of work. There is no easy way to become involved in public policy formulation. It will require extensive writing, reading of legislation, analyzing of legislation, and creating written comment. At some point in the administrator's career, he or she may be asked to make presentations before governmental bodies, legislative entities, etc. Usually this represents the culmination of many years of active involvement in the development of public policy. This form of leadership will not only be personally satisfying for the individual, but it will put the administrator's facility or service in a leadership position with other comparable services. It will afford that administrator a glimpse into the future, and make him or her better able to plan for the future.

Additionally, the interaction in the public policy sector will enable the practicing administrator to better understand regulations, laws, and other public policy edicts that have a direct impact on this operation. This enhanced understanding will not only allow one to work better within the system, but will give the administrator the necessary staff training tools to provide proper supervision to key professional employees.

REFORM: THE BY-WORD IN PUBLIC POLICY

Probably the most important element in contemporary public policy is the reform of the Medicare and Medicaid program. Although these programs have had almost two decades of operation, there are still problems in financing and inadequacies in the service programs that have existed since their inception in the mid '60s. Integral with these two problem areas is a massive effort to reduce both current expenditures and the explosion of future expenditures.

Medicaid unfortunately is not a single program but a collection of programs that vary by state. Poor families and children, the elderly and other functionally impaired individuals, and the mentally retarded and developmentally disabled are the three major population groups now funded by Medicaid resources. Very often the poor, elderly, disabled, and mentally impaired are lumped together, since basic health care needs are fundamentally different from social health needs of other people, for example those with chronic functional impairment. Due to categorical restrictions in benefit determination, a large percentage of the nation's poor are ineligible for Medicaid benefits. It has been suggested that a significant public policy change would be to establish a national eligibility standard based on a predetermined nationwide poverty level. Therefore health care services would be based on a uniform financial need program. The public policy change that would create a nationally homogeneous Medicaid Program has been labelled by some as a national primary care program which would also include the establishment of a primary care and preventive health benefit package that would be appropriate to augment the care of the poor. On the other hand, the states would be relegated the responsibility of providing social support needs to the functionally impaired elderly disabled and to the mentally retarded and developmentally disabled. Other elements of this major national policy change would be prepaid capitated financing using primary care physicians as gate keepers in cost control and utilization. Because the federal government finances and administers this facet of the program, they should also be responsible for eligibility determination, competitive bidding for services contracting with eligible providers and reimbursement monitoring. States could be able to administer these programs under special contract with the federal government.

Career Development

MANAGEMENT IN THE HISTORICAL PERSPECTIVE

Up through the '50s, the "management" leadership of any health facility was most likely a physician. With the exception of leadership that stemmed from a religious orientation, the physician dominated management in most facilities. In the early '50s, when the "nursing home" was primarily a small dwelling converted for the long term care of the elderly, management consisted of the ownership of these facilities. At the start of the '60s there were no particular professional tracks, training programs, or required certifications. In the early expansion of the nursing home industry, a most eclectic group of people was in charge of administration. Many were people with no health experience who got into the field because they had some relationship with the ownership. In the nonprofit and governmental sectors, social workers and religious leaders were the administrators of most of the facilities. During the early '60s, when the first signs of the nursing home systems' expansion became evident, key organizations were founded that could be considered the point of departure for long term care administration as a profession.

In 1962, the American Nursing Home Association and the American Association of Homes for the Aged were founded. The latter represented the nonprofit sector and the former the proprietary or profit making sector. Also in this year, the American College of Health Care Administrators, then known as the American College of Nursing Home Administrators, was founded. Thus the effort to professionalize long term care administration began.

Throughout the ensuing years, each of these organizations has contributed significantly to the advancement of both the knowledge of the subject of administration in this field, and the enhancement of the career potential of a long term care administrator. The American College of Health Administrators, which currently has a membership of over 6,000 long term care administrators, has as its goal furthering the professional component of providing care and acting as an advocate for the profession through coordinated action, communication and fellowship. The College, as it is known, has a heavy involvement in training, education and upgrading of professional standards. It was responsible for developing the first code of ethics in this field.

While these two associations, AAJA and AHCA (or trade associations as some refer to them), were directed to enhance their sector of the long term

care field, the American College directed itself more specifically to enhancing the profession, through the setting of standards, research, education,
and as I mentioned before in the development of a code of ethics. The
ACHCA also has a referral service for job opportunities. The social security
amendments of 1967, signed into law in January 1968 by President
Johnson, became the major impetus for the upgrading and evolution of the
nursing home administrator as a professional. The following quote from a
statement made by Senator Edward Kennedy in the hearings aptly describes
the role of the nursing home administrator.

> This information has convinced me that the operator or administrator
> of a nursing home is the key person in assuring that the care received
> by a nursing home resident is a very high quality. The operator, is,
> after all, a man who hires and fires a staff; the man who orders the
> food; the man who schedules visits by physicians; and in general, the
> man who *sets the standards by which each individual nursing home
> operates.*

Further on in this same testimony, the senator stated

> that states presently require the licensing of doctors, of dentists,
> lawyers, architects, of engineers and of other professionals as well.
> This licensing process ensures that the public interest in receiving ser-
> vices, meaning some minimum requirements of quality, are met. Since
> nursing home operators are directly responsible for assuring day to
> day that their residents receive the medical care they need. It is my
> firm belief that the operator should be licensed by the states in the
> same way as doctors, dentists and lawyers.

As part of the same deliberations during the development of these amendments, the senate committee on financing stated "licensure of administrator
should result in increased professionalization and enhanced status for those
charged with the important responsibility of caring for hundreds of
thousands of older Americans. A licensed nursing home administrator will
become clearly identified as a health professional."

The amendments called for the creation of a national advisory council on
nursing home administration to oversee the implementation of this component of the amendments, and a contract to the professional examination
service for the preparation of questions for a nursing home administrators
licensure examination was awarded by the U.S. Public Health Service. Even
though the Federal regulations included descriptions of a core curriculum
and standards for nursing home licensure, there were still many differences
on the state level because of wide variations of definitions and vocabulary.
The American College of Nursing Home Administrators developed definitions that were adopted by other national organizations and these have
become the definitions used in licensing and education and all other aspects
of development of the nursing home field.

Even though we do have a uniform set of definitions and federal standards, states may still vary by requiring Bachelor's Degrees or other specific job oriented experiences. Most require a completion of a nursing home administrator examination and the completion of either an academic internship or an administrative training program under the direction of a qualified preceptor. Additionally, most states require continuing education in order to retain the license. The licensure examination is provided by the National Association of Boards of Examiners for Nursing Home Administrators (NAB) with the assistance of the professional examination service. The exam relates to general administration, resident care, and federal rules and regulations.

There are some states that currently require a bachelor's degree to sit for the examination and may require a master's degree in the near future. The masters may be in health care administration or a related field.

In the early '60s, when asking how to learn to run a nursing home, most prospective administrators were directed to learn by speaking to practicing administrators. A decade later, all of the states were under a federal mandate to license nursing home administrators and intermediate care facilities. One of the surprise results of the first round of examinations was the elimination of a large number of individuals who were unable to pass the examination. An analysis of those who were successful in passing the examination indicated that a minority of those had bachelor degrees, and even a smaller minority had masters degrees. During the ensuing years these ratios would change. A similar study done in the early '80s would show that a majority had bachelor degrees, and a significant number of people had masters degrees in health or hospital administration or a related field.

In 1973 the Association of University Programs in Hospital Administration conducted the first national symposium on long term care administrator education. At that time most of the academic programs involved in administrator education taught a 100 hour education for nursing home administrators which was funded by the federal government. By the mid-'70s with the disappearance of these federal funds, the courses disappeared. Five years later, AUPHA conducted a similar symposium on long term care and noted that 72 educational institutions prepared students for this field. Forty-eight of these schools indicated that they provided long term care administration level at the associate, baccalaureate or at the masters degree level.

Currently there is no distinct category for schools that specialize in long term care administration. The schools that train people for long term care administration, emphasize of course the nursing home and intermediate care facility.

At the symposium it became quite clear that there were diverse viewpoints on the specific curricula that would be appropriate for the nursing home administrator. From these deliberations came many recommendations that filtered through the system, and ultimately impacted the academic curricula, examination questions, and substance of the continuing education programs.

MEETING THE NEEDS OF THE CONTINUUM

Despite all this activity generated to upgrade the administration of the skilled nursing and intermediate care facility, little attention has been given to meeting the administrative needs of the other components of the continuum.

Senior housing probably is an exception to this statement. The federal government has developed a sophisticated housing managers training program and has required its implementation throughout the country for public housing managers.

There are numerous examples of attempt to license or certify the administrator of residential care facilities for the elderly, but at this point there are no states which require this licensing or certification to run these non-medical facilities.

If you were to take the 20,000 skilled nursing and intermediate care administrative positions and augment them by the numbers of administrators of adult day health care, nutrition sites, transportation services, and home health programs, you would find the numbers of management positions in the field of long term care (when viewed in this manner) to be extraordinarily large.

MANAGEMENT FOR THE CONTINUUM

Unfortunately, the management needs for the various parts of the continuum have not attracted very much attention. Yet, on close analysis, we find that many programs fail or do not function in an optimal manner because of this lack of management capability.

Consistently, we find these programs administered by professionals from other disciplines who have worked their way up from the field, and have had little benefit of or interest in management training. Professionals who run these organizations usually address their management proficiency in a secondary way, often relegating "management and paperwork details" to other individuals in their organization. This author believes that each component of the continuum of care should have professional administration that follows the same guiding principles which created the nursing home administrator field. It is my opinion that each one of these forms a subcomponent of the long term care field as a profession, and there should be either training programs that deal with the components of the continuum specifically, allowing the certification in a number of areas, or that there be one long term care administrator license.

THE CASE FOR THE GENERIC LONG TERM CARE
ADMINISTRATOR LICENSE

The idea of a long term care license that will train an individual to manage any or all parts of the continuum of care interests me, and I think its day has come. No longer can we address the professional competency of only segments of the continuum, when it is quite clear that the other components of the continuum are equally as valuable, as complex, and in need of professional administration. It is my opinion that the attitudes of the various disciplines that supply the trained professionals who currently run these organizations should be compromised in view of the need of the entire system to upgrade itself.

I propose that, rather than have individual licenses, the concept of the nursing home license should be expanded to cover all of the services of the continuum, and to embody this into an amendment of the Social Security Act similar to that which took place in 1967.

The diverse professional groups that feed into the long term care system would have to be agreeable to this proposal. However, probably the biggest barrier would be individuals in the field who may not view this licensure as necessary. Some of the artificial barriers that have been put up to this advancement in professionalism have come from the owners and administrators of residential care homes for the elderly. They feel that the costs incurred in licensure, certification and training are not economically feasible. Other professional groups do not want to ally themselves with the nursing home profession. Still others feel that management is a subordinate function to their particular method of running an agency. All of these barriers must be overcome. The creation of a generic long term care administrative license throughout the country would be a major force in unifying long term care and the most significant step forward to improve the overall quality of services being rendered to the elderly population.

CAREERS IN LONG TERM CARE

As we have discussed, the field of serving the elderly expanded substantially during the '70s and will continue to do so in terms of complexity as the elderly aging population expands. It is of utmost importance for public policy makers to recognize the need to upgrade the management of all of these service entities. And it is very important that academia recognizes long term care as a viable growing career opportunity for the many undergraduate students who are seeking to enter the field of human services.

The opening up of an entire new professional structure allowing for appropriately trained younger people at the entry level and the upgrading of the capabilities of mid-career professionals is an imperative for the '80s. It is important that we do not wait until there is obvious degradation of the system or specific service elements to embark upon this licensure. Already there are signs of "decay" if one were to believe the media, and it is certainly not too late to recognize that an injection of professionalism, high level academic training, and coalescence of divergent professional approaches is vitally needed for the long term care system of the future.

Bibliography

Alex Comfort, *"The Process of Aging,"* Signet Science Library, 1964.

Luvernn Cunningham and William Gebhart, "Leadership: The Science and the Art Today," F. E. Peacock Publishers, Inc., 1973.

Olget Knopf, M.D., *"Successful Aging: The Facts and Fallacies of Growing Old,"* The Viking Press, 1975.

Robert Kavanaugh, *"Facing Death,"* Nash Publishing Company, 1972.

Richard Lampbert, Allen Heston, "Political Consequences of Aging," *Annals of the American Academy of Political Science,* Volume 415, 1974.

Allen Goldstein, M.D., *"Age, Patients and Long Term Care Facility: A Staff Manual,"* National Institute of Health, Section on Mental Health of the Aging, 1973.

Joan Krauskopf, *"Advocacy for the Aging,"* West Publishing Company, 1983.

The Manager Foundation, *"Toward Understanding Therapeutic Care: A Training Guide for In-Service Education in the Psychosocial Components in Long Term Care,"* contract HRA30-76-0281 Health Resources Administration, Division of Long Term Care, Department of Health, Education and Welfare.

Morris Rockstein, Marvin Sussman, *"Nutrition and Longevity,"* Academic Press, New York 1976.

Frank Moss and Val Hanlamandaris, *"Too Old, Too Sick, Too Bad,"* Aspen Publication, 1977.

Ron Kayne, Ph.D., *"Drugs and the Elderly,"* Ethel Percy Andrus Gerontological Center, 1978.

Joan Birchenall, RN, M.Ed., and Marilee Streight, RN, BSN, *"Care of the Older Adult,* J. B. Lippincott and Co., 1973.

Irwin Rausch, Maria Perper, *"Resident Care Management System,"* CBI Publishing Company, 1980.

Linda Horn and Elmin Griesel, *"Nursing Home: A Citizens Action Guide,"* Beacons Press, Boston, 1977.

Richard Lam and Associates, *"Community Survival for Long Term Care Patients,"* Jossey Bass Publishers, 1976.

Elaine Brody and Contributors, *"A Social Work Guide for Long Term Care Facilities,"* National Institute of Mental Health, 1974.

Carolyn B. Stevens, *"Special Needs of Long Term Care Patients,"* J.B. Lippincott and Company, 1974.

Sandra H. Johnson, *"Long Term Care and the Law,"* National Health Publishing, 1983.

Suzanne Haynes, Ph.D., Manning Feinleib, Doctor of Public Health,

"Epidemiology of Aging," U.S. Department of Health and Human Resources, 1983.

Cyril Brickfield, Alfred Miller, *"The Legal Rights of the Elderly,"* Practicing Law Institute, CR-3180, 1974.

Bernice Neugarten, Robert Havighurst, *"Social Policy, Social Ethics, and the Aging Society,"* University of Chicago Press, Committee on Human Development, 1976.

E.V. Cowdry, Ph.D. and Franz Steinberg, M.D., *"Care of the Geriatric Patient,"* The C.V. Mosby Company, 1971.

Index